COLOUR GUIDE

D1647507

	07/03/08	
2 APR 1999	-2 APR 2008	
4 MAY 1999		
14 MAY 1999		
02 JUL 1999	-4 MAR 2009	
	1 9 JUL 2010	
15 SEP 2000	2 7 APR 2011	
	1 0 DEC 2018	
28 MAR 2001		
1 1 MAY 2002		
1 2 JUL 2002		
1 1 SEP 2002		
2 7 JUL 2004		
1 5 JUL 2005		

LIVINGSTONE

EDINBURGH LONDON MAD
SAN FRANCISCO TOKYO 19

CHURCHILL LIVINGSTONE
Medical Division of Pearson Professional Limited

Distributed in the United States of America by
Churchill Livingstone Inc., 650 Avenue of the
Americas, New York, N.Y. 10011, and by
associated companies, branches and
representatives throughout the world.

First Colour Guide edition 1992
Second Colour Guide edition 1997

ISBN 0 443 05807 5

British Library Cataloguing in Publication Data
A catalogue record for this book is available from
the British Library.

**Library of Congress Cataloging in Publication
Data**
A catalog record for this book is available from
the Library of Congress.

Medical knowledge is constantly
changing. As new information
becomes available, changes in
treatment, procedures, equipment
and the use of drugs become
necessary. The editors/authors/
contributors and the publishers
have, as far as it is possible,
taken care to ensure that the
information given in this text is
accurate and up to date.
However, readers are strongly
advised to confirm that the
information, especially with
regard to drug usage, complies
with current legislation and
standards of practice.

The
publisher's
policy is to use
**paper manufactured
from sustainable forests**

For Churchill Livingstone

Publisher: Michael Parkinson
Project editor: James Dale
Production controller:
Kay Hunston
Design direction: Erik Bigland

Produced by Longman Asia Limited, Hong Kong
SWTC/01

Acknowledgements

We are extremely grateful to the following colleagues for providing us with illustrations: Stephen Bryan (Figs 4 & 7); Paul Butler (Figs 14, 30, 37, 39, 45, 46, 49, 51, 53, 60, 61, 64, 65, 67, 68, 69, 71, 76, 78, 82, 85, 86, 89, 90, 94, 140, 141, 142, 143, 145, 148, 150, 151, 153, 157, 158, 159, 164, 166, 171, 172, 176, 181); Rex Dawson (Figs 55 & 183); Richard Frackowiak (Fig. 101); Bill Gibb (Figs 99, 100, 102); Cathinka Guldberg (Fig. 41); Bob Ham (Fig. 56); Ivor Levy (Figs 8, 9, 10, 11, 12); Christian Lueck (Fig. 26); John Monson (Fig. 70); Nick Murray (Fig. 36); Julia Newton (Figs 29, 75, 79, 88, 160 & 162); David Perry (Fig. 147); Donald Scott (Figs 72, 73, 92, 172 & 174); Elizabeth Shaw (Figs 80, 83 & 84); David Spalton (Figs 5 & 6); Roger Sutton (Fig. 74); P. K. Thomas (Figs 114 & 115); Ed Thompson (Fig. 93).

We acknowledge the dedication of Ian Berle and the staff of the Medical Photography Department of the Royal London Hospital who were responsible for the majority of the photographs. The manuscript has been typed and retyped by Linda Self, to whom we wish to express our thanks and appreciation.

P. T.
M. S.
C. K.

Contents

Cranial nerve I—olfactory nerve

The olfactory nerve relays the sense of smell from receptor cells in the mucous membrane of the nasal cavity to the olfactory tract via the cribriform plate.

Clinical tests

Various standard odours are placed in turn adjacent to each nostril whilst the other is occluded. The patient is asked to sniff and identify the odour.

Lesions

These include local disturbances of the nasal cavity and damage to the nerve due to head trauma. Other causes include tumours, e.g. meningiomas of the olfactory groove, and multiple sclerosis.

Cranial nerve II—optic nerve

The optic nerve is a purely sensory nerve, transmitting visual information from the retina to different visual centres in the brain.

Clinical tests

Measure the visual acuity, and record colour vision in each eye. Confrontation testing of the visual fields is often sufficient to determine the presence of hemianopias, quadrantanopias and central or paracentral scotomas. Careful ophthalmoscopic examination of the fundus is essential (Fig. 1). Normal variants such as a large optic cup (Fig. 2) and medullated retinal nerve fibres (Fig. 3) must be distinguished. The most common abnormalities are those due to hypertension (silver wiring, AV nipping, hard exudates and flame haemorrhages; Fig. 4) and diabetes mellitus (dot haemorrhages, soft exudates and new vessel formation; Fig. 5).

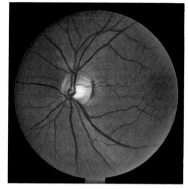

Fig. 1 A normal fundus and optic disc.

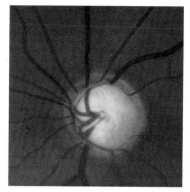

Fig. 2 Large optic cup. May be normal variant or due to glaucoma.

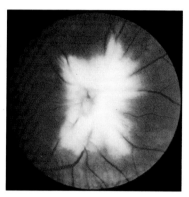

Fig. 3 Medullated retinal nerve fibres.

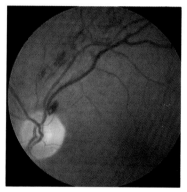

Fig. 4 Hypertensive retinopathy.

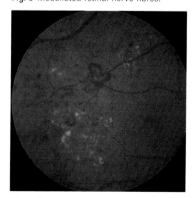

Fig. 5 Diabetic retinopathy.

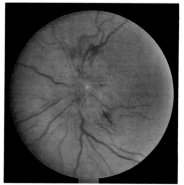

Fig. 6 Papilloedema due to raised intracranial pressure.

Optic disc swelling

This may signify serious underlying neurological or systemic disease. Important causes of optic disc swelling include the following.

Papilloedema: (see Fig. 6, p. 2) not associated with visual loss when due to raised intracranial pressure, except at the end stage if left untreated. Common causes are intracranial tumours and hydrocephalus.

Pseudopapilloedema: usually due to the presence of small calcified bodies (drusen) at the disc margin (Fig. 7), or to small optic disc with tortuous peripapillary vessels.

Optic neuritis: local causes of disc oedema are distinguished from papilloedema by the presence of visual loss in the early stages. They include inflammation (papillitis), demyelination (multiple sclerosis), vascular lesions (central retinal vein occlusions), tumours (optic nerve meningiomas) and infiltrations (e.g. sarcoid and lymphomas).

Optic atrophy

Optic atrophy leads to a pale disc and may result primarily from disease of the optic nerve or chiasma, without any intervening visible changes (Fig. 8). It may be due to multiple sclerosis, trauma, nerve compression by tumour (which may give rise to optociliary shunts, Fig. 9), neurosyphilis or toxic causes such as alcohol, drugs (e.g. ethambutol) and tobacco. In secondary optic atrophy the disc margins are blurred; this follows papillitis, chronic papilloedema and periarteritis.

Vascular disturbances

The central retinal artery may be occluded, e.g. by embolus (Fig. 10), or the central retinal vein (Fig. 11) may thrombose. Anterior ischaemic optic neuropathy may be due to giant cell arteritis (Fig. 12), but more commonly is atherosclerotic.

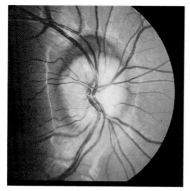

Fig. 7 Pseudopapilloedema, with small refractive bodies at disc margin (drusen).

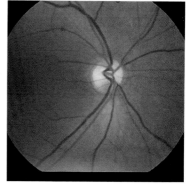

Fig. 8 Optic disc atrophy. Note disc pallor due to glaucoma.

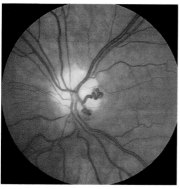

Fig. 9 Optociliary shunts—usually due to optic nerve meningioma.

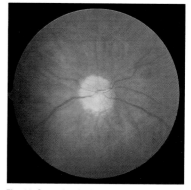

Fig. 10 Central retinal artery occlusion.

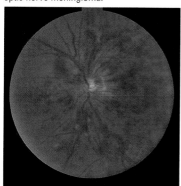

Fig. 11 Central retinal vein occlusion.

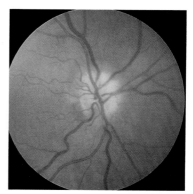

Fig. 12 Anterior ischaemic optic neuropathy due to giant cell arteritis.

Proptosis is the pathological forward displacement of one or both eyes.

Differential diagnosis

The most common cause of acquired proptosis is dysthyroid eye disease. This may present unilaterally or bilaterally (exophthalmos). The most frequent accompanying abnormality is lid retraction (Fig. 13). Systemic features of thyrotoxicosis are often present, although the condition may be found in a euthyroid patient. Other causes of unilateral proptosis are:
- *orbital tumours*: primary such as haemangiomas, dermoids, tumours of the optic nerve, e.g. meningiomas or gliomas (Fig. 14); secondary, e.g. due to carcinoma of the breast
- *carotico-cavernous fistula* (Fig. 15)
- *idiopathic orbital inflammation* (pseudotumours) or *orbital cellulitis*.

Investigations

If the cause is not apparent clinically, CT scanning of the orbit is the most useful investigation. This will reveal orbital tumours and enlargement of the extraocular muscles in dysthyroid eye disease. Carotid angiography may be necessary in a suspected carotico-cavernous fistula.

Management

Dysthyroid eye disease: treatment of thyrotoxicosis if present; steroids and orbital decompression if the optic nerve is compromised.

Carotico-cavernous fistula: may spontaneously resolve, or may require closure by induced thrombosis of the cavernous sinus.

Tumour: surgical excision, except with optic nerve meningiomas and optic gliomas of childhood.

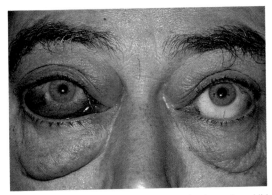

Fig. 13 Thyroid eye disease, causing proptosis, chemosis and lid oedema.

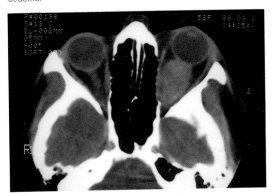

Fig. 14 CT scan showing left optic nerve glioma.

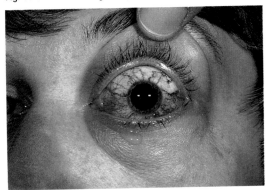

Fig. 15 Proptosis caused by a carotico-cavernous fistula. A loud bruit was heard over the globe.

3 / The pupil

The pupil diameter is controlled by the autonomic nervous system. The pupilloconstrictor fibres are controlled by the parasympathetic division, and pupillodilator fibres by the sympathetic division.

Lesions

Argyll Robertson pupils

This pupillary abnormality is the hallmark of a late syphilitic infection of the central nervous system (Fig. 16). The pupils are small and irregular in outline, showing an impaired or absent direct light response, although the near response is intact. Such dissociation of the near pupillary responses to light may also occur in diabetes mellitus, or with midbrain tumours, when the pupils are of normal size or dilated.

Horner syndrome

This syndrome is due to a lesion anywhere along the sympathetic pathway to the pupil. It is characterized by a small ipsilateral pupil, mild ptosis (Fig. 17) and ipsilateral facial anhidrosis. There is an intact direct light reflex. The topical diagnosis of Horner syndrome is dependent on accompanying signs and symptoms, but the most common cause of an isolated Horner syndrome is a malignancy. This is usually bronchogenic or breast carcinoma involving sympathetic fibres at the chest apex (Pancoast's tumour).

Tonic (Holmes–Adie) pupil syndrome

In this syndrome, due to a parasympathetic lesion in the ciliary ganglion, the involved pupil is larger than its fellow and shows a poor or absent light reaction (Fig. 18). With accommodative effort it slowly constricts. When the near reflex is relaxed, the pupil dilates very slowly. This pupillary syndrome is benign, and is most common in young women. It is often associated with diminished deep tendon reflexes.

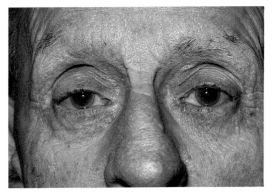

Fig. 16 Argyll Robertson pupils.

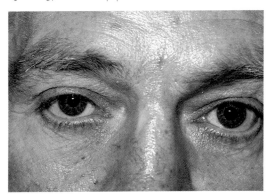

Fig. 17 Horner syndrome (right) with mild ptosis. Note the right pupil is smaller than the left.

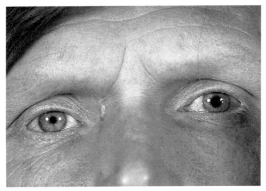

Fig. 18 Tonic (Holmes–Adie) pupil (left). Dilated pupil fails to respond to light.

4 / Cranial nerve III—oculomotor nerve

The oculomotor nerve supplies the levator palpebrae superioris, superior rectus, inferior rectus, medial rectus and inferior oblique ocular muscles. It also carries the pupilloconstrictor (parasympathetic) fibres.

Clinical features

A complete third nerve palsy presents with a complete ptosis (Fig. 19), fixed dilated pupil (Fig. 20) and ocular motor palsy, except for abduction (Fig. 21).

Lesions

Vascular: a brainstem infarction which usually also involves pyramidal and cerebellar pathways, resulting in a contralateral hemiplegia and ipsilateral cerebellar ataxia. In the subarachnoid space the nerve lies adjacent to the posterior communicating artery (PCA). An aneurysm (see Fig. 57, p. 36) of this vessel, often associated with ipsilateral periorbital pain, is the most common cause of an oculomotor palsy with pupillary involvement. Aneurysms in the cavernous sinus involve the fourth, fifth and sixth cranial nerves to varying degrees, in addition to the oculomotor nerve. In patients over the age of 55 years, a sudden onset pupil-sparing third nerve palsy is usually associated with evidence of vascular disease, such as atherosclerosis, hypertension or diabetes mellitus. The lesion is in the oculomotor nerve itself.

Neoplastic: the oculomotor nerve may be involved by tumours at many different sites, usually metastatic or by direct spread from a nasopharyngeal carcinoma.

Infective: caused by basal meningitis such as tuberculosis.

Demyelinating: as part of multiple sclerosis.

Trauma: head injuries may cause avulsion of the nerve as it emerges from the brain stem.

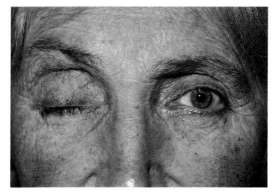

Fig. 19 Complete right ptosis in oculomotor nerve palsy.

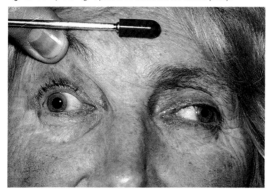

Fig. 20 Dilated right pupil and failure of adduction in oculomotor nerve palsy.

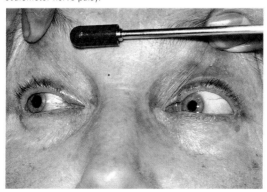

Fig. 21 Oculomotor nerve palsy. Normal right abduction reveals normally innervated lateral rectus muscle.

Cranial nerve IV—trochlear nerve

The trochlear nerve innervates the superior oblique muscle which produces depression and intorsion of the globe in the adducted position.

Lesions

The most common causes for an isolated trochlear nerve palsy are head trauma, ischaemia associated with atherosclerosis or diabetes mellitus, and neoplasms.

Cranial nerve VI—abducens nerve

The abducens nerve innervates the lateral rectus muscle which abducts the eye. It has a particularly long intracranial course.

Lesions

Congenital: Duane syndrome due to aplasia of the abducens nucleus (Figs 22 & 23).

Vascular: a sixth nerve lesion when associated with ipsilateral facial palsy and contralateral hemiparesis suggests brainstem infarction. In the cavernous sinus the sixth nerve may be damaged by carotico-cavernous fistula, aneurysm of the internal carotid or by thrombosis. Here the third, fourth and fifth cranial nerves are also often involved.

Neoplastic: tumours of the cavernous sinus and orbital apex, invasion of skull base and chordomas.

Infective: middle ear disease spreading to petrous apex, and meningitis—especially tuberculous.

Demyelinating: as part of multiple sclerosis (Fig. 24).

Trauma: skull base fractures.

Raised intracranial pressure: may cause a palsy which is a false localizing sign.

Mimickers: isolated ocular motor palsies can be mimicked by thyroid eye disease and myasthenia gravis. Appropriate tests must be performed to exclude them.

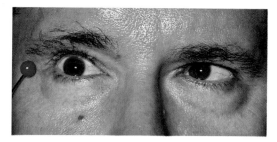

Fig. 22 Gaze to the right shows failed abduction in Duane syndrome (right).

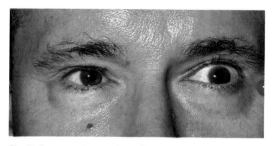

Fig. 23 Duane syndrome (right). Gaze to the left shows narrowing of palpebral fissure with intact adduction.

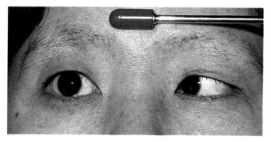

Fig. 24 Failure of abduction of the right eye in abducens nerve palsy caused by multiple sclerosis.

Horizontal gaze palsies

As well as containing the motor neurons innervating the ipsilateral lateral rectus, the abducens nucleus contains neurons which connect to the medial rectus subnucleus of the contralateral third nerve nucleus. These axons pass along the medial longitudinal fasciculus. A lesion of the abducens nucleus therefore results in an *ipsilateral conjugate gaze palsy*. A lesion of the medial longitudinal fasciculus gives rise to a failure of adduction of the ipsilateral eye; this is called an *internuclear ophthalmoplegia* (INO, Fig. 25).

Clinical tests   In a possible INO, observe the abducting eye, which usually shows a few beats of nystagmus. Always test horizontal rapid saccadic eye movements, since in a partial INO only slow adduction may be observed, without a paresis (Fig. 26).

Lesions   *Vascular:*   pontine infarction or haemorrhage.

Neoplastic: usually pontine metastases.

Demyelinating: the most common cause; bilateral INOs are frequently seen in multiple sclerosis.

Vertical gaze palsies

Lesions of the neural centres for vertical gaze, which lie in the midbrain rostral to the oculomotor nucleus, usually result in up and down gaze paralysis. Also look for other features of rostral midbrain dysfunction (Parinaud syndrome). These include lid retraction, dilated pupils which react poorly to light and impairment of upward gaze (Fig. 27). Attempted upward gaze may also result in convergence–retraction nystagmus, in which the eyes make converging nystagmoid movements associated with apparent retraction of the globes. The most common cause is a pinealoma.

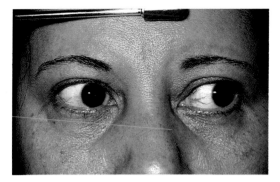

Fig. 25 A right internuclear ophthalmoplegia—impaired adduction of right eye with abducting nystagmus of left eye.

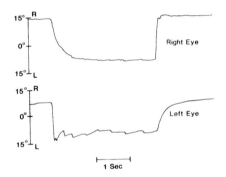

Fig. 26 An eye movement recording of the same patient in Figure 25. Note slowed adduction of the right eye, i.e. during gaze towards the left.

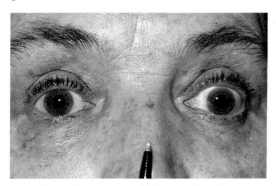

Fig. 27 Failure of upward gaze with lid retraction in Parinaud syndrome.

The trigeminal nerve is a mixed sensory and motor nerve, and is the largest of all the cranial nerves. It conveys sensation from the face and scalp to the vertex, and from the oronasal mucous membranes and teeth. It provides the motor supply to the muscles of mastication.

Clinical tests

When testing facial sensation with pin and touch, remember that the ophthalmic division spreads back to the vertex and that the angle of the jaw is supplied by the second cervical dermatome. Pay special attention to the corneal reflex, which should be elicited from the inferolateral quadrant. Look for wasting of temporalis and masseter muscles, test the power of jaw opening and watch for deviation. Never forget the jaw jerk.

Lesions

Vascular: as part of posterior inferior cerebellar artery occlusion, lateral pontine syndrome (Fig. 28), aneurysms, arteriovenous malformations (AVMs) or ectasia of the basilar artery in the posterior fossa and of the carotid in the cavernous sinus.

Neoplastic: trigeminal neurinoma (Fig. 30), posterior fossa tumours, invasion of the skull base, tumours of cerebellopontine angle, cavernous sinus and orbital apex.

Infective: middle ear disease spreading to the petrous apex, herpes simplex and zoster infections (usually ophthalmic, Fig. 29).

Demyelinating: as part of multiple sclerosis.

Trauma: skull base fractures.

Tic douloureux (trigeminal neuralgia)
Highly distinctive brief episodes of severe lancinating unilateral facial pain, usually in either maxillary (nose/eye) or in mandibular (mouth/ear) divisions, triggered by touch, shaving, chewing, talking and yawning. Slightly more common in women with onset in the mid-50s. Responds to carbamazepine, or neurovascular decompression of the V nerve in the posterior fossa.

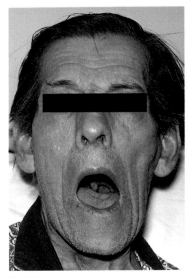

Fig. 28 Left lateral pontine syndrome.

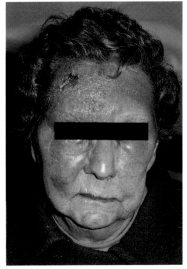

Fig. 29 Herpes zoster ophthalmicus.

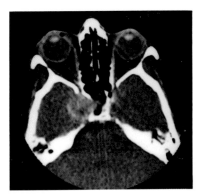

Fig. 30 Right trigeminal neurinoma as seen in CT scan.

8 / Cranial nerve VII—facial nerve

The facial nerve is a mixed sensory and motor nerve. It conveys taste sensation from the anterior two-thirds of the tongue, and provides the motor supply to the muscles of facial expression.

Clinical features

The upper half of the face receives a bilateral supranuclear supply; thus an upper motor neuron lesion principally produces movement impairment of the lower half of the contralateral face (Fig. 31). A lower motor neuron lesion involves the whole of one side of the face equally.

Lesions

Bell's palsy: (Figs 32 & 33) the most common disorder of the facial nerve. It affects the sexes equally and occurs at all ages. Diabetes mellitus and hypertension may predispose. There is acute onset, often with a prodromal ache behind the ear and subjective facial numbness. Hyperacusis and taste impairment may be present in a proximal lesion. Steroids are helpful if seen early and the lesion is fairly complete. About 80% recover in the first month. In more severe cases, aberrant regeneration may lead to crocodile tears and jaw-winking. Consider sarcoid, lymphoma and Guillain–Barré syndrome if the condition is bilateral.

Ramsey–Hunt syndrome: a herpes zoster infection of the geniculate ganglion, in which facial palsy is associated with vesicles in the external auditory meatus and in the oropharynx. The V, VIII and IX cranial nerves may also be involved.

Hemifacial spasm: (Fig. 34) usually starts locally around one eye and then spreads. The condition is induced by facial movement, and is usually idiopathic, although it may be caused by structural lesions within the posterior fossa, cerebellopontine angle and around the skull base. The condition is responsive to local injections of botulinum toxin into the overactive facial muscle.

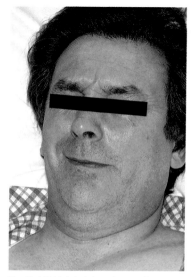

Fig. 31 Mild left facial weakness of upper motor neuron type.

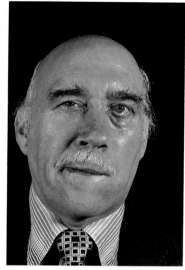

Fig. 32 Left Bell's palsy: 'smile'.

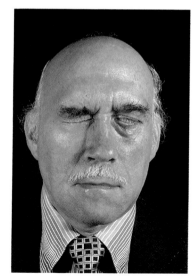

Fig. 33 Left Bell's palsy: 'screw up your eyes'.

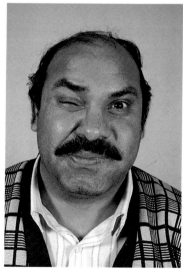

Fig. 34 Right hemifacial spasm.

The VIII cranial nerve is purely sensory and has two parts:
- the *cochlear nerve* (from the organ of Corti) subserves hearing
- the *vestibular nerve* (from the semicircular canals and otoliths) is concerned with balance and body orientation.

Clinical tests

Hearing may be tested at the bedside either with a ticking watch or with whispers. Tuning fork tests (Rinne and Weber, with a 512 Hz tuning fork) distinguish conductive deafness due to external and middle ear disease from sensorineural or nerve deafness. If the main complaint is of vertigo, then positional testing, with the patient rapidly moving from the sitting position to lying supine with the neck extended and turned to one side, may induce the symptoms and can occasionally produce nystagmus (Fig. 181, p. 118). This is typical of benign paroxysmal positional vertigo. Formal audiometry (Fig. 35), brainstem auditory evoked potentials (Fig. 36) and caloric tests are usually helpful.

Lesions

Nerve deafness may be due to the following.

Acoustic neuroma: (Fig. 37) progressive deafness associated with tinnitus, impaired balance, facial pain or paresis, with later cerebellar and long tract signs. If bilateral or familial, consider neurofibromatosis, type 2 (NF2).

Menière's disease: intense bouts of vertigo and vomiting associated with tinnitus and deafness, and superimposed upon a background of progressive unilateral hearing loss which often predates the first attack. Onset is typically over the age of 50 years.

Ototoxic drugs: aminoglycosides, quinine and aspirin.

Other causes of vertigo: benign positional vertigo, acute vestibular neuronitis, vascular disease, multiple sclerosis and temporal lobe epilepsy.

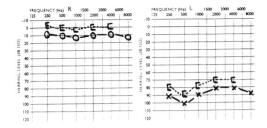

Fig. 35 Audiogram showing left-sided deafness of sensorineural type.

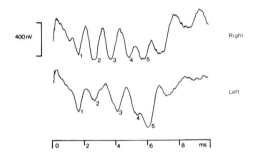

Fig. 36 Brainstem auditory evoked potentials showing left-sided delay of waves 3–5.

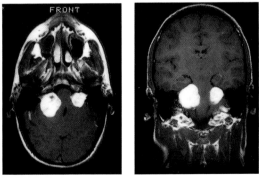

Fig. 37 Bilateral acoustic neuromas seen in MRI brain scan with axial view (left) and coronal view (right).

The glossopharyngeal (IX) and vagus (X) nerves arise from the medulla and are mixed. The spinal accessory nerve (XI) is purely motor. The IX nerve conveys superficial sensibility from the oropharynx, taste sensation from the posterior third of the tongue, and innervates the carotid body. It provides the motor supply to the stylopharyngeus, and is secretomotor to the parotid. The X nerve conveys sensation from a small area of skin in the ear and contains visceral afferents from the aortic arch and respiratory and alimentary tracts. Somatic motor fibres supply the larynx, pharynx and palate; visceral cholinergic motor fibres innervate the hearts, bronchi and gastrointestinal tract. The XI nerve provides the motor supply to the sternomastoid (Fig. 38) and the upper part of the trapezius muscle.

Clinical tests

Touch and pain sensation over the oropharynx should be tested (IX). Look for a hoarse voice with bovine cough, nasal speech, drooping of the soft palate with uvular deviation and loss of gag reflex (X). Test for wasting (Fig. 38), and power of the sternomastoid and trapezius muscles (XI).

Lesions

- IX, X and XI nerves may be affected within the medulla and upper cervical cord by motor neuron disease, polio, syringomyelia and vascular disease.
- These nerves are often involved together in the jugular foramen by neurofibroma, meningioma, granulomas, glomus tumours (Fig. 39), metastatic carcinoma and vertebral artery aneurysms.
- X and XI may be damaged in the neck by trauma, usually knife wounds.
- X may also be affected in the chest, by mediastinal tumours, lung cancer and aneurysms of the aortic arch.

Glossopharyngeal neuralgia
Severe lancinating pain (trigeminal neuralgia) is experienced in the throat whenever food is swallowed. Carbamazepine is of help.

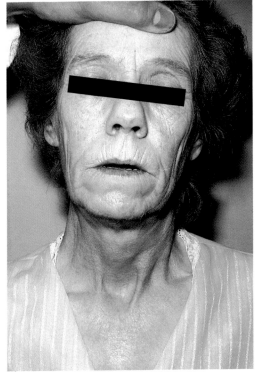

Fig. 38 Wasting of right sternomastoid muscle.

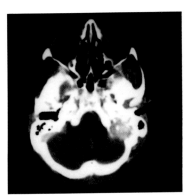

Fig. 39 Typical left glomus tumour seen in CT brain scan.

The hypoglossal nerve is purely motor. It emerges between the pyramid and the olive, and exits through the hypoglossal canal. It innervates the muscles of the tongue, principally the genioglossus.

Clinical features

Wasting and fasciculation of the affected side of the tongue characterize a lower motor neuron lesion. On protrusion, the tongue deviates to the weak side. In upper motor neuron lesions, the tongue is small, spastic and moves only slowly from side to side.

Lesions

The XII nerve is usually damaged in conjunction with other cranial nerves, though rarely it may be affected alone. This occurs in the medial medullary syndrome (in association with a crossed hemiplegia) and in diseases of the skull base—flattening or platybasia, Paget's disease and neoplastic invasion (usually metastatic, Fig. 40). Extracranial causes include cervical lymphadenopathy (again usually malignant) where there is often an associated Horner syndrome.

Bulbar palsy

This is the result of a lower motor neuron-type of weakness of the muscles supplied by the V, VII, IX, X, XI and XII cranial nerves. Features include difficulty in chewing, bifacial weakness and weakness of the muscles of the pharynx and larynx (dysphagia and dysphonia), the sternomastoid and trapezii, and the tongue (dysarthria). Causes include poliomyelitis, diphtheria, syringobulbia and motor neuron disease.

Pseudobulbar palsy

Bulbar palsy should be distinguished from *pseudobulbar palsy*. This syndrome results from bilateral upper motor neuron lesions interrupting the corticobulbar pathways. Spastic weakness of the bulbar musculature results, often with additional emotional lability. Causes include multiple lacunar strokes, multiple sclerosis and motor neuron disease. Video fluoroscopy is a useful investigation (Fig. 41).

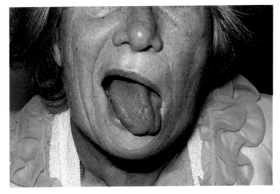

Fig. 40 Weakness in the left side of the tongue causes it to protrude to the left. In this case the cause was a secondary deposit in the skull base.

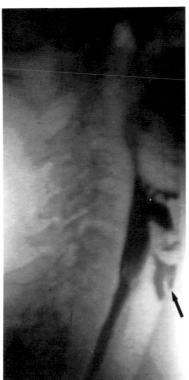

Fig. 41 Video fluoroscopy. Note pharyngeal pooling and tracheal aspiration.

Transient ischaemic attacks (TIAs) are defined as a neurological deficit lasting less than 24 h due to a focal reduction in cerebral blood flow. TIAs are a common symptom with an incidence of 2.2 per 1000 per year in the elderly (>65 years) population.

Aetiology

The most common cause is embolic. Emboli either come from atheromatous lesions, typically at the origin of the internal carotid artery, or from the heart.

Clinical features

Carotid territory TIAs
These are of two main types:
- *Amaurosis fugax* is characterized by a monocular loss of vision. Ophthalmoscopy during an attack may reveal a retinal embolus (Fig. 42). The episode usually lasts 5–30 min with complete return of vision.
- *Involvement of the middle cerebral artery* may lead to weakness, numbness and heaviness of the contralateral arm and leg; *involvement of the dominant hemisphere* can cause dysphasia.

Vertebrobasilar territory TIAs
The most common symptoms are vertigo, diplopia, dysarthria, facial paraesthesiae or visual disturbances, bilateral weakness or sensory disturbance and drop attacks. Cardiac emboli may also cause skin lesions (Fig. 43).

Investigations

- *Blood tests*: haemoglobin, platelets, clotting screen, glucose, serology and lipids.
- *ECG and echocardiogram*: to exclude cardiac dysrhythmia and valvular defect.
- *Doppler ultrasound*: a good non-invasive method of determining carotid artery stenosis.
- *Cerebral angiography* (Fig. 44).

Management

Aspirin, 300 mg daily, has been shown to reduce the risk of a subsequent completed stroke if the carotid stenosis is less than 70%. For tighter stenoses carotid and arterectomy is more effective than aspirin.

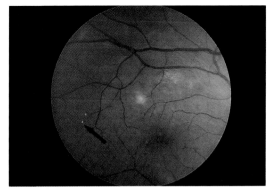

Fig. 42 Amaurosis fugax. Fundus photograph showing artery embolus (arrow).

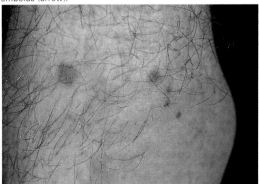

Fig. 43 Purpuric skin lesions due to emboli from a diseased mitral valve.

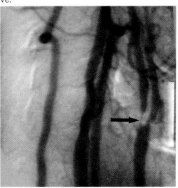

Fig. 44 Internal carotid stenosis. Digital subtraction angiogram showing stenosis of the left internal carotid artery (arrow).

13 / Cerebral thrombosis

Incidence

The frequency of cerebral thrombosis increases with age, and has an overall incidence of between 1 and 2 cases per 1000 of the population per annum. Hypertension and diabetes mellitus often pre-exist and there is usually evidence of vascular disease in other parts of the body, e.g. angina pectoris and intermittent claudication.

Investigations

Investigation should concentrate on screening for possible risk factors such as polycythemia, hyperlipidaemia and diabetes mellitus in the hope of preventing further episodes. CT scans reveal the extent of cerebral infarction (Figs 45 & 46) and may show luxury perfusion (Fig. 47). In younger patients cerebral angiography may be indicated, particularly if the neurological deficit is not too severe.

Management

There is no specific treatment to improve or hasten recovery after cerebral infarction. The blood pressure should be monitored, but hypertension, other than that of the malignant type, should not be urgently treated since it is often reactive and necessary to maintain cerebral perfusion in the area around the infarction. It will settle to normal levels in at least 40% of cases after 3 weeks. Physical therapy should be instituted as soon as possible after onset to prevent complications such as subluxation of the shoulder and deep vein thrombosis. Continuation of physical therapy, together with occupational therapy, is essential to restore the patient to maximum achievable mobility.

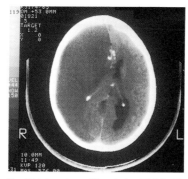

Fig. 45 Internal carotid occlusion (right). CT scan shows low density in anterior and middle cerebral artery distributions.

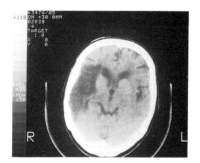

Fig. 46 Middle cerebral artery occlusion (right). CT scan shows more restricted low density in region around the Sylvian fissure.

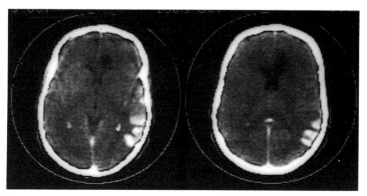

Fig. 47 Luxury perfusion on axial CT scans after injection of contrast (left middle cerebral artery distribution).

Cerebral haemorrhage is usually associated with small micro-aneurysms (Charcot–Bouchard aneurysms) located in deep cerebral structures such as the thalamus, striatum, pons and cerebellum.

Clinical features

Spontaneous rupture of the micro-aneurysm may occur causing haemorrhage, and producing a severe headache with rapid depression of the conscious level. If the haemorrhages rupture into the ventricles, the patient usually complains of severe headaches as in a subarachnoid haemorrhage (Fig. 48). Less severe haemorrhages result in clinical signs appropriate to their location; for example in a thalamic haemorrhage there is a contralateral hemiplegia with sensory loss and a disorder of vertical eye movements.

Clinically, it is difficult to differentiate intracranial haemorrhage from infarction, but CT scanning has proved most effective in differentiating between the two conditions (Fig. 49). A cerebellar haemorrhage is of particular concern since the patient may initially present with brainstem signs attributed to infarction and a few days later rapidly deteriorate due to coning (Fig. 50), causing progressive brainstem distortion, leading to failure of the vital centres and death unless the haemorrhage is evacuated.

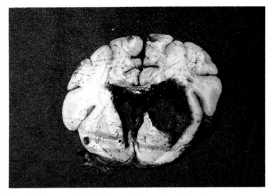

Fig. 48 Intraventricular haemorrhage at post-mortem.

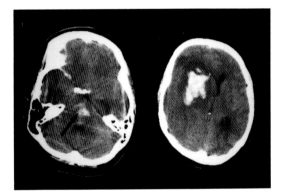

Fig. 49 Large right intracerebral haemorrhage with secondary pontine bleed (arrow) as seen in axial CT scans.

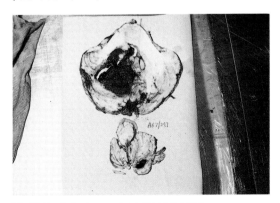

Fig. 50 Cerebellar haemorrhage at post-mortem.

Developmental abnormalities can result in abnormal connections between the arterial and venous systems. They vary in size, tending to expand over the years, and can occur anywhere within the brain.

Clinical features

AVMs usually present between the ages of 16 and 30 years as a result of rupture, but occasionally they are seen with focal seizures. The initial rupture usually leads to both subarachnoid and intraparenchymal haemorrhage, the latter resulting in focal neurological deficits. The consequences of rupture are not usually as severe as after berry aneurysm rupture, the mortality being around 10%.

Management

Once the feeding vessels have been determined by angiography (Fig. 51), surgical treatment by extirpation of the whole malformation is feasible only if it is superficially placed (Fig. 52). Embolization therapy and stereotactic radiotherapy are also proving useful. Some angiomas do not appear on MRI (Fig. 53) but may be revealed by angiography. Other causes of intracranial haemorrhage are trauma, bleeding diatheses, cerebral tumours and septic emboli from infective endocarditis.

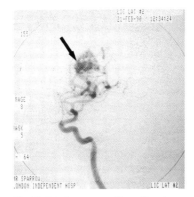

Fig. 51 Arteriovenous malformation. An angiogram showing a tangled mass of abnormal vessels (arrow).

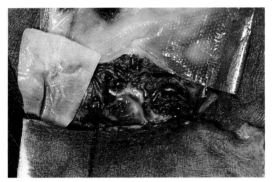

Fig. 52 Per-operative view of a large AVM.

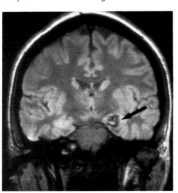

Fig. 53 Cavernous angioma (arrow) revealed on an MRI scan in medial aspect of right temporal lobe.

Emboli, usually from the heart or an atheromatous plaque, pass into the cerebral circulation causing an obstruction at some point which results in ischaemic infarction.

Aetiology

- *Cardiac:* chronic atrial fibrillation (due to atherosclerotic or rheumatic heart disease with embolism from thrombus in the atrial appendage), valvular heart disease (Fig. 54) and atrial myxoma (Fig. 55).
- *Non-cardiac:* includes atherosclerosis of aorta and carotid arteries, thrombus in pulmonary veins, and fat, tumour and air embolism.

Management

General medical management is required in the acute phase, followed by physical therapy and rehabilitation. During this time, investigations to identify the source of the embolus are carried out.

If a cardiac source is found, anticoagulation is the treatment of choice in preventing further emboli. Initially, heparinization followed by warfarin is recommended.

An atheromatous plaque in the internal carotid artery is best dealt with by carotid endarterectomy (Fig. 56). Endarterectomy is indicated when the plaque causes luminal stenosis of 70% or more (see Fig. 44, p. 26).

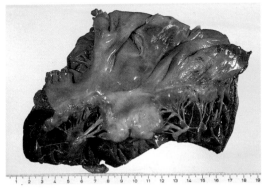

Fig. 54 Mitral valve leaflet prolapse.

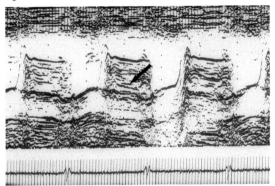

Fig. 55 Echocardiogram showing features of a left atrial myxoma.
Note multiple echoes from within left atrium (arrow).

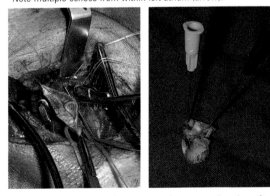

Fig. 56 Internal carotid endarterectomy. A per-operative view after
the atheromatous plaque has been removed (left). The dissected
plaque from the same case (right).

Approximately 5% of cerebrovascular accidents are due to subarachnoid haemorrhage in which rupture of a blood vessel results in extravasated blood leaking into the subarachnoid space. It is usually due to rupture of an intracranial berry aneurysm, but may occur from a cerebral angioma or the extension of an intracerebral haemorrhage into the subarachnoid space. Berry aneurysms are usually located on the circle of Willis or at a bifurcation of one of the cerebral arteries, and are considered to be due to a congenital defect of the media (Figs 57 & 58). The mortality from the initial haemorrhage is about 40%, with the risk of re-bleeding gradually declining with time.

Clinical features

These include sudden onset of severe excruciating headache, vomiting and photophobia. There may be almost instantaneous loss of consciousness. Clinical examination reveals neck stiffness (Kernig sign) and sometimes a subhyaloid haemorrhage (Fig. 59). Focal neurological signs may be due to expansion of the aneurysm, e.g. an oculomotor nerve palsy due to a posterior communicating aneurysm or an associated intracranial haematoma.

Investigations

The clinical diagnosis is confirmed by CT scanning (Fig. 60). Lumbar puncture is necessary if the scan is normal. Confirmation of the location of the aneurysm is made by angiography performed soon after onset.

Management

Treatment rather depends on the clinical state of the patient, with conservative management if coma persists, or neurosurgical clipping of the aneurysm if the patient's condition allows.

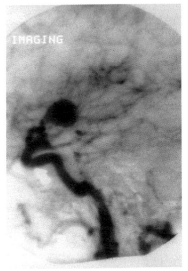

Fig. 57 A carotid angiogram shows a large anterior communicating artery aneurysm.

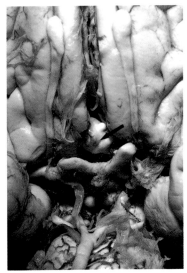

Fig. 58 Post-mortem specimen revealing large anterior communicating artery aneurysm (arrow) between the two cerebral hemispheres.

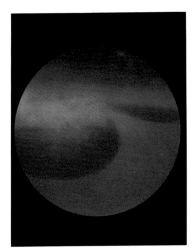

Fig. 59 Subhyaloid haemorrhage. Fundoscopic view after a large subarachnoid haemorrhage.

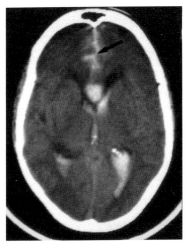

Fig. 60 Subarachnoid haemorrhage. A CT scan shows blood (high density) in the ventricles and interhemispheric fissure.

In adults, brain tumours represent 2% of all malignancies. Half are primary tumours of the brain, its coverings and the pituitary gland; the other half are metastases. Certain genetic disorders, e.g. neurofibromatosis, predispose to brain tumours.

Clinical features

Brain tumours present either with focal disturbances or raised intracranial pressure. Large tumours, regardless of their location, cause progressive mental slowing, forgetfulness and personality change. About 10% of patients with epilepsy commencing after age 20 years have brain tumours, especially meningioma, astrocytoma (Figs 61 & 62), metastases (Fig. 63) or lymphoma (Fig. 64).

Seizures may be focal or generalized, but occur only with supratentorial tumours, whether intrinsic or extrinsic to the brain. Progressive focal abnormalities, e.g. hemiparesis, visual disturbance, aphasia or cerebellar ataxia are characteristic. Raised intracranial pressure causes headache, vomiting and papilloedema. Headache is typically present on waking in the morning, and relieved 30–60 min after getting out of bed, but may be more persistent. Posterior fossa tumours, especially in childhood, present with raised intracranial pressure. ➡

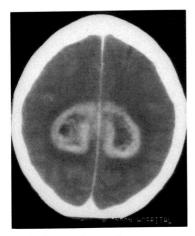

Fig. 61 Corpus callosum glioma (glioblastoma).

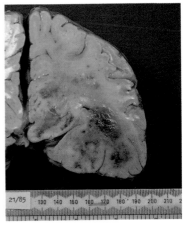

Fig. 62 Glioma of left temporal lobe with swelling of left hemisphere.

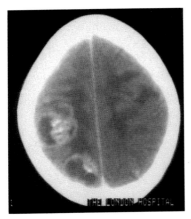

Fig. 63 Multiple metastases in both hemispheres.

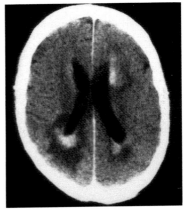

Fig. 64 Lymphoma with multiple lesions in the deep white matter.

Types

Gliomas: intrinsic neuro-epithelial tumours arising from the glial-supporting tissue of the brain. They are always locally invasive and may be cystic; they often undergo malignant transformation.

Astrocytomas: in the corpus callosum (Fig. 61, p. 38) produce marked personality changes, with frontal lobe deficits. The temporal lobe (Fig. 62, p. 38) is a common location of astrocytomas, often causing partial seizures with a prominent olfactory and gustatory aura. The focal mass lesion may lead to uncal herniation, causing drowsiness and ipsilateral third nerve palsy.

Lymphoma: (Fig. 64, p. 38) occurs as a primary tumour or as part of a generalized process. It is especially common in AIDS.

Metastases: (Fig. 63, p. 38) frequently multiple and usually located at the grey/white matter junction. Tumours of the lung, breast, kidney and thyroid, and melanomas are common primary tumours.

Meningiomas: (Figs 65 & 66) common and usually located at the convexity of the brain, on the sphenoid wing, in the parasellar region, in the lateral ventricles, in the posterior fossa or in the orbit. They are slow-growing and may be very large, causing a stroke-like presentation or leading to recurrent focal or generalized seizures. Sometimes small cortical meningiomas may present with epilepsy. If technically feasible, surgical removal should be complete.

Colloid cysts: (Fig. 67) dense, cystic tumours containing proteinaceous fluid, usually found in the third ventricle. They may lead to headache due to intermittent hydrocephalus.

Medulloblastoma: (Fig. 68) a radiosensitive malignant tumour, usually found in the cerebellum in children, that may metastasize widely within the CSF pathways.

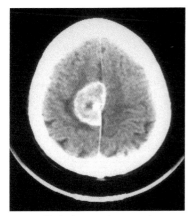

Fig. 65 Meningioma at the convexity.

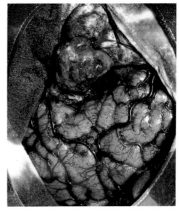

Fig. 66 Operative view of meningioma on parietal surface of brain.

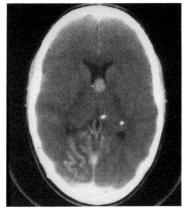

Fig. 67 Colloid cyst in third ventricle, appearing as a high density lesion. There is infarction in the right occipital region with hyperperfusion of the ischaemic region.

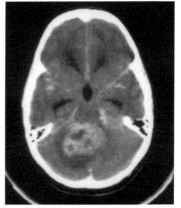

Fig. 68 Medulloblastoma in vermis of cerebellum of a child.

Pituitary tumours

Pituitary adenomas may be functioning, non-functioning, or inappropriately functioning. They may cause mass effects on neighbouring structures, or may be functioning micro-adenomas.

Large tumours erode the pituitary fossa (Fig. 69) and damage the optic chiasm, leading to bitemporal hemianopia, optic atrophy and panhypopituitarism. Functioning tumours are usually small, especially prolactinomas which cause infertility, loss of libido and galactorrhoea with amenorrhoea. Acromegaly (Fig. 70) occurs when there is uncontrolled secretion of growth hormone. CT or MR scanning is useful for accurately delineating the pituitary fossa and the extent of lateral and superior growth of pituitary tumours (Fig. 71).

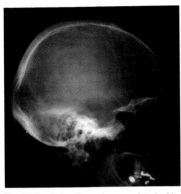

Fig. 69 Eroded sella turcica associated with large chromophobe adenoma of pituitary.

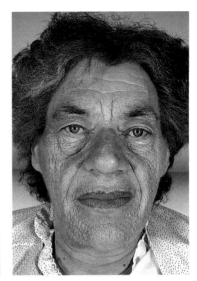

Fig. 70 Acromegaly.

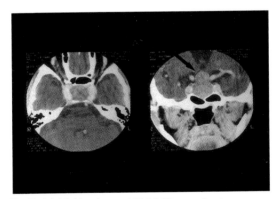

Fig. 71 Axial (left) and coronal (right) CT scans showing expansion of the pituitary fossa by a tumour. Note the suprasellar extension (arrow).

Epilepsy is a tendency to have seizures: it is not a disease. A seizure is a condition in which the normal orderly pattern of cerebral neuronal discharge is acutely deranged, usually only briefly.

Classification

Generalized epilepsy—without focal onset

Tonic/clonic (grand mal or major) attacks: begin with a cry, transient limb stiffening and, often, incontinence. Jerking next occurs which slows down over a minute; there may be tongue biting. Typically, the patient experiences post-ictal drowsiness for an hour.

Absence (petit mal or minor) attacks: brief blank spells characterized by staring eyes with dilated pupils, eyelid fluttering, facial and limb jerks, fumbling of the hands, chewing and lip-smacking movements. The EEG is characteristic with three-per-second high voltage spike and wave discharges (Fig. 72).

Partial (focal) epilepsy—with focal onset

Simple (without altered consciousness): may be motor (adversive or a Jacksonian march), sensory (visual, auditory, olfactory and vertiginous) or autonomic (visceral) in type.

Complex (with altered consciousness): typified by 'temporal lobe epilepsy' with memory and mood changes, déjà vu, hallucinations and automatisms. Both types of partial seizure may secondarily generalize.

Clinical tests

- *EEG* (Fig. 73): resting and sleep records.
- A number of *blood tests* including sugar, WR and calcium, as well as ECG in younger patients.
- *Cranial CT*: particularly in older age groups (>20 years of age) or with a clear focal onset on EEG. MR imaging is more sensitive, particularly if surgery is being considered.
- *Ambulatory EEG* or *video-telemetry* in diagnostic difficulties.

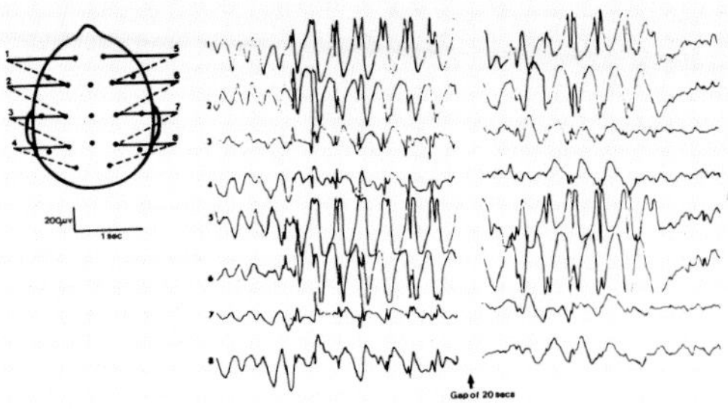

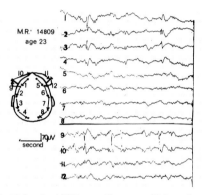

Fig. 72 Three-per-second spike and wave typical of petit mal epilepsy.

Fig. 73 Interictal EEG record in temporal lobe epilepsy showing left temporal complexes (Channels 1–4, 9, 10).

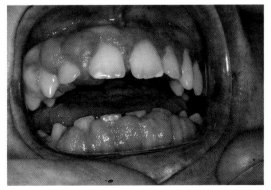

Fig. 74 Unwanted effect of phenytoin treatment: gum hyperplasia.

Aetiology	*Symptomatic epilepsy:* in infants, consider congenital malformations and metabolic abnormalities; in children, consider perinatal anoxia, birth injury and phakomatoses (Figs 75–78). In adults, alcohol and drug intoxication and withdrawal, tumours, vascular and degenerative disease may be present. In all age groups, consider trauma and infections, particularly meningitis.
	Idiopathic epilepsy: presents in adolescence and is often associated with a positive family history of epilepsy, a past history of febrile fits and petit mal attacks, and photosensitivity on EEG.
Management	Be sure of the diagnosis—functional attacks known as pseudoseizures are common. Do not treat a single seizure unless the EEG is very abnormal. With multiple seizures use a reputable first line drug, such as sodium valproate, phenytoin (Fig. 74, p. 44) and carbamazepine, as monotherapy at a minimum effective dose. If frequent seizures persist, use blood levels to optimize the dose, check compliance and exclude toxicity. Add further drugs such as lamotrogine, vigabactin or gabapentin only exceptionally. Surgical excision may be considered in a very few cases after full imaging studies and more sophisticated EEG. Metabolism of the contraceptive pill is increased by phenytoin and carbamazepine; use a high oestrogen pill or two mini pills daily. Carbamazepine is the safest drug to take through a pregnancy. In the UK, patients holding driving licences should be advised they have an obligation to inform the Driver and Vehicle Licensing Agency about attacks of altered consciousness, whether these be epileptic or not.

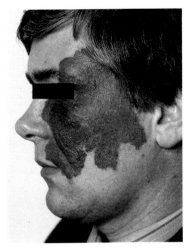

Fig. 75 Sturge–Weber naevus is often associated with epilepsy.

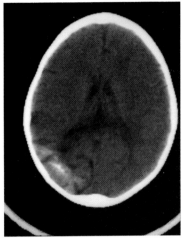

Fig. 76 Calcification and focal atrophy of parieto-occipital cortex in Sturge–Weber syndrome as seen on CT scan.

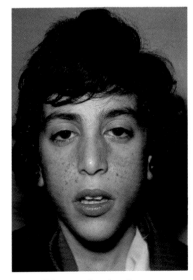

Fig. 77 Tuberose sclerosis: adenoma sebaceum.

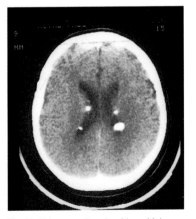

Fig. 78 Tuberose sclerosis with multiple paraventricular calcified masses (tubers) as seen on CT scan.

Bacterial meningitis

Aetiology

The three most common causative agents are:
- *Neisseria meningitidis* (meningococcus): young adults; may occur in epidemics.
- *Streptococcus pneumoniae* (pneumococcus): older age group; think of sinus and middle ear disease.
- *Haemophilus influenzae*: usually children under six years.

Clinical features

These include fever with headache, photophobia, neck and back stiffness with later drowsiness and vomiting. Occasionally, fits may occur in young children, and a typical rash (Fig. 79) with meningococcal disease. Findings include nuchal rigidity and positive Kernig sign.

Clinical tests

Cranial CT is taken prior to lumbar puncture (LP) only when there is papilloedema or clear focal features, including altered consciousness. At LP, turbid CSF under increased pressure (200–300 mm), raised white cell count, typically 1000–10 000 per mm^3 and usually more than 80% polymorphs. Raised protein between 1 and 5 g/l and depressed sugar, below 2.5 mmol/l. Gram stain may be positive (Fig. 80).

Management

A third generation cephalosporin is administered until Gram stain result, then appropriate antibiotics are given for 2 weeks. Steroids are in general unhelpful, and intrathecal therapy is dangerous. In meningococcal disease, consider chemoprophylaxis for very close contacts only.

Complications

These include deafness, optic atrophy, hemiplegia, cortical vein or sinus thrombosis, hydrocephalus and subdural effusions and empyema (Fig. 81). If meningitis is recurrent, consider the presence of cranial or spinal defects, either congenital or traumatic in type, and diseases associated with immunosuppression.

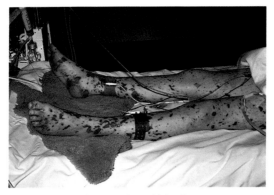

Fig. 79 Typical meningococcal petechial rash.

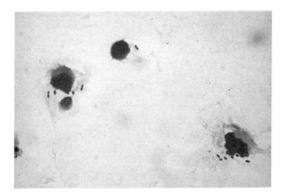

Fig. 80 Gram-positive diplococci—pneumococcal meningitis.

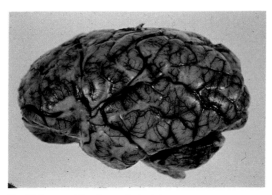

Fig. 81 Pus overlying the cortical sulci.

Tuberculous meningitis

Clinical features

The condition is characterized by an insidious presentation with fever, headache, lethargy, anorexia, weight loss, intellectual decline and personality change. Fits and vomiting occur in young children.

Clinical tests

Cranial CT shows basal enhancement (Fig. 82). There is colourless CSF under slightly raised pressure (200–250 mm) at LP, 50–400 white cells, mainly lymphocytes, raised protein between 1–2 g/l and either normal or depressed glucose level. The main differential diagnoses include fungal and malignant meningitis. Ziehl–Neelsen staining may show acid-fast bacilli (Fig. 83).

Management

This includes isoniazid (with pyridoxine supplements), rifampicin and pyrazinamide for 12 months. Pyrazinamide may be discontinued earlier. Steroids are more useful, particularly when there is clouding of consciousness or spinal block. Complications include inappropriate ADH secretion, hydrocephalus and tuberculoma formation (Fig. 85, p. 52).

Fungal meningitis

Clinical features

Fungal meningitis is most frequently associated with immunocompromised patients, organ transplantation, malignancy, steroid treatment or connective tissue diseases. The most common is cryptococcal disease, though *Candida* and mucormycosis may occur.

Clinical tests

CSF shows less than 300 white cells, usually a mix of polymorphs and lymphocytes, raised protein though rarely more than 1.5 g/l and normal or slightly depressed glucose level. India-ink preparations may show the fungal cells (Fig. 84).

Management

In cryptococcal disease, amphotericin B and flucytosine may be used, though the mortality rate in general is high.

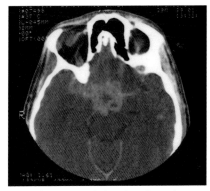

Fig. 82 Enhancement in basal exudates of tuberculous meningitis as shown in CT scan.

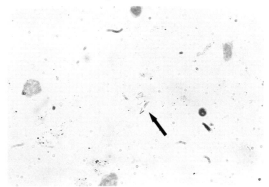

Fig. 83 Acid-fast bacilli (cluster in centre) in Ziehl–Neelsen preparation.

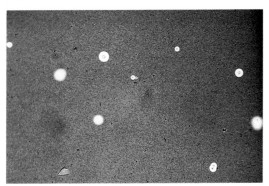

Fig. 84 Cryptococcal cells outlined by the carbon in India-ink preparation.

Cerebral abscess

Aetiology

A cerebral abscess can result from direct spread of infection from paranasal sinuses and teeth (frontal lobe involvement) or from middle ear and mastoid disease (temporal lobe and cerebellum). Alternatively, it can be blood borne from lung disease (abscess, bronchiectasis or TB, Fig. 85), endocarditis or cyanotic congenital heart disease. Subdural empyema may also be caused by trauma and neurosurgery. Any organism may be involved; the most common are streptococci, staphylococci and anaerobes.

Clinical features

These include raised intracranial pressure (headache, drowsiness and vomiting), focal signs and seizures with or without fever, and varying degrees of meningeal irritation.

Clinical tests

Cranial CT or MRI shows a hypodense lesion with mass effect and ring enhancement (Fig. 86). EEG may be helpful in showing focal delta waves. Lumbar puncture is contraindicated. Sinus and chest X-rays and appropriate cultures should be performed.

Management

Aggressive regime of broad-spectrum antibiotics should be administered in the first instance, with anticonvulsants and steroids. Assess regularly with serial CT or MRI. If unresponsive, consider surgical aspiration or excision. Multiloculated abscesses and intraventricular rupture both worsen prognosis (Fig. 87).

Viral meningitis

Viral meningitis is usually caused by the mumps virus or one of the enteroviruses (echovirus/coxsackie).

Clinical features

A mild illness with headache, photophobia, malaise and neck stiffness, often preceded by fever and chills. Clear CSF under increased pressure typically yields 10–1000 lymphocytes, a protein rarely above 1 g/l and a normal glucose concentration.

Management

No treatment is required and a full recovery occurs over some days.

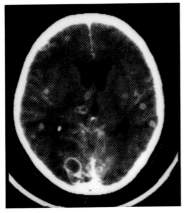

Fig. 85 Multiple tuberculomas as seen on CT scan.

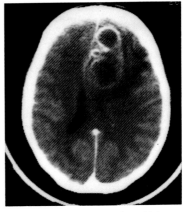

Fig. 86 Large multiloculated frontal lobe abscess showing ring enhancement and midline shift as seen on CT scan.

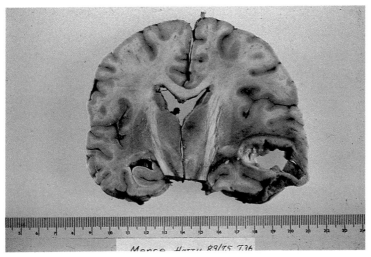

Fig. 87 Chronic, thick-walled temporal lobe abscess post-mortem.

Viral encephalitis

Herpes simplex virus (type 1 usually) is the most common cause (Fig. 88).

Clinical features

The meningeal symptoms are generally less impressive than in bacterial meningitis and are accompanied by progressive depression of consciousness, focal features, seizures and abnormal movements. Cranial CT initially shows swelling and low density within both temporal lobes, often with scattered haemorrhages, and later there is focal atrophy (Fig. 89). The CSF is often under greatly increased pressure, contains up to 1000 lymphocytes, with a normal or slightly reduced glucose and an elevated protein concentration between 1–1.5 g/l. The EEG reveals background slowing and characteristic bitemporal periodic complexes at regular 2–3 s intervals. Blood and CSF serology is occasionally rewarding. Rarely, the virus can be isolated from CSF or cultured from brain biopsies.

Management

Treat with I/V acyclovir at first clinical suspicion and steroids to control raised pressure. Anticonvulsants can be used if necessary. Mortality remains at 30%, and 60% of the survivors are left with permanent deficits, usually amnesia and difficult seizures.

Other viral infections

Progressive multifocal leucoencephalopathy (PML) is another viral cerebral infection (Fig. 90). It is caused by one of the papovaviruses and is seen mostly in the immunocompromised. The infection is rare, but is particularly associated with HIV infection as a manifestation of AIDS.

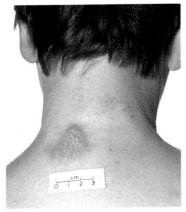

Fig. 88 Typical herpetic lesion on neck.

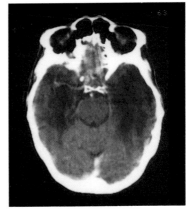

Fig. 89 Bitemporal low density in old herpes simplex encephalitis seen on CT scan.

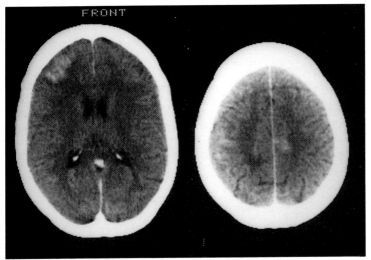

Fig. 90 PML seen on CT scan. Diffuse low density change in white matter with small haemorrhage in the right frontal area.

21 / Multiple sclerosis

Multiple sclerosis is a demyelinating disease characterized by neurological symptoms and signs indicative of two or more lesions disseminated within the CNS, both in time and space.

Prevalence

Females show a greater prevalence than males, with a ratio of 1.8:1. The age of onset is 10–60, and is typically in the early 30s.

Aetiology

The cause is unknown. There is an increasing risk with increasing latitude; for example, the condition has an incidence of one case per 100000 on the equator, and 140 per 100000 in Scotland. There is a familial predisposition. An association with HLA-DR2 exists, and there is a more loose relationship with a number of autoimmune diseases.

Clinical features

Typical modes of presentation include optic neuritis (Fig. 91), brainstem features (vertigo, diplopia, nystagmus and ataxia), spastic paraparesis and sphincter disturbance with impotence. Suggestive single features include trigeminal neuralgia, facial myokymia, Lhermitte sign (limb tingling on neck flexion) and Uhthoff (exacerbation of symptoms with heat and exercise) phenomena. The course is either relapsing and remitting, often with a phase of secondary progression or primarily progressive (particularly if over the age of 40). ➡

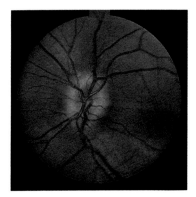

Fig. 91 Mild optic disc swelling in acute optic neuritis.

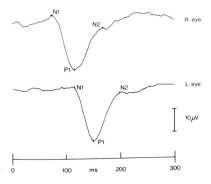

Fig. 92 Delayed left eye visual-evoked potential (P1).

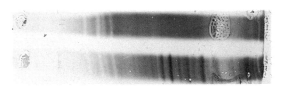

Fig. 93 CSF isoelectric focusing from normal (above) and MS patient (below). Oligoclonal bands (dark vertical lines on bottom trace) of IgG are seen.

Clinical tests

There is no diagnostic test; the diagnosis is clinical. Evoked potentials—visual (Fig. 92, p. 56), brain-stem and somatosensory—may demonstrate a sub-clinical lesion. CSF examination may show up to 50 mononuclear cells. The protein may be slightly increased though rarely above 1 g/l, and the sugar is always normal. The proportion of IgG is usually raised and oligoclonal bands may be present on electrophoresis (Fig. 93, p. 56). Cranial CT is usually normal though may show generalized atrophy; acute plaques are occasionally seen to enhance after a high dose of contrast. MR imaging often shows multiple sub-clinical lesions, typically in a periventricular location (Figs 94 & 95) and within the brainstem and cerebellum. The core pathological lesion seen in acute MS is perivascular cuffing with mononuclear cells and lymphocytes (Fig. 96).

Management

There is no cure for the disease. Steroids are traditionally used to shorten exacerbations. Rest is important. Fatigue may be helped by amantadine or pemoline. Urinary urgency usually responds to oxybutylin, though intermittent self-catheterization may eventually be necessary. Limb spasticity may be treated with baclofen or dantrolene, and pain often responds to tricyclics or anticonvulsants. Impotence can be helped by intracavernous papaverine injections. β–interferon therapy reduces the risk of relapses in relapsing/remitting MS and may improve the prognosis regarding disability.

Other demyelinating diseases include central pontine myelinolysis and Marchiafava–Bignami disease.

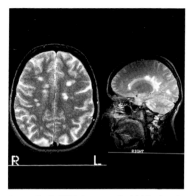

Fig. 94 Brain MRI shows typical high signal periventricular lesions in MS.

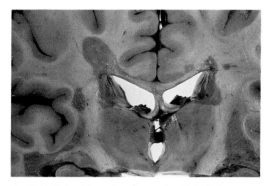

Fig. 95 Multiple white matter plaques at post-mortem.

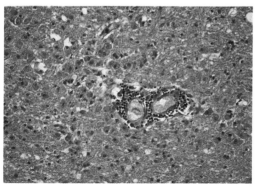

Fig. 96 Mononuclear cell perivascular cuffing in acute MS.

Idiopathic Parkinson's disease

Clinical features

The four classic features are tremor, rigidity, bradykinesia and impaired postural reflexes. The tremor is usually present at rest, and has a frequency of 4–6 Hz. Passive flexion and extension of the wrist or elbow usually reveals a recurrent catch followed by a relaxation; this is called cogwheel rigidity. The most disabling feature of the disease is bradykinesia. There is delay in initiation of movement which is itself slow. Fine movements such as writing (Fig. 97) and doing up buttons become increasingly difficult. Walking is slowed, with small steps (shuffling gait), difficulty in turning and failure to swing the arms. The posture is flexed, with the head and back bowed and the arms held partially flexed (Fig. 98). The face shows a typical immobility—the 'Parkinsonian mask'.

Management

In the early stages, treatment is with anticholinergic drugs; benzhexol or orphenadine may be sufficient and of particular benefit for tremor. When the patient becomes more severely affected, dopamine replacement using the precursor L-dopa, combined with a peripheral dopa decarboxylase inhibitor, should be used. After treatment for 5 years, about 50% of patients develop motor fluctuations, called the on–off syndrome. Commonly, the duration of action of the L-dopa gets progressively shorter (the wearing off effect), or there may be sudden swings between profound immobility and dyskinesia. Dopaminergic drugs, e.g. pergolide, are used at this stage of the disease. Stereotactic lesioning of the pallidum may also be beneficial in the later stages in relieving tremor. Subthalamic stimulation may relieve bradykinesia in intractable cases. ➡

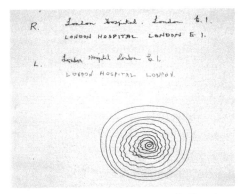

Fig. 97 The handwriting of a patient with Parkinson's disease. This shows micrographia and the tremulous spiral.

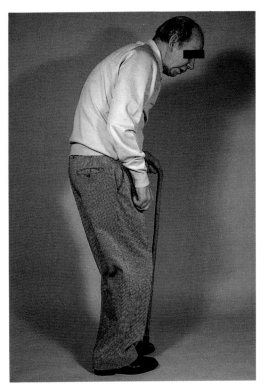

Fig. 98 Parkinson's disease showing typical flexed posture in an advanced case.

Parkinson's disease is the most common disorder involving the basal ganglia, with a prevalence of about 1 in 1000 of the population. The main pathological abnormality is degeneration of the substantia nigra (Figs 99 & 100). This leads to a depletion of dopamine in the corpus striatum (Fig. 101). The remaining cells show a characteristic inclusion, the Lewy body (Fig. 102, p. 64). Although most cases are of the idiopathic form, Parkinsonian features result from drugs, especially neuroleptics, and may rarely result from infections as seen in encephalitis lethargica in the 1920s. The toxic agent 1-methyl-4-phenyl-1, 2, 5, 6-tetrahydropyridine (MPTP), a pethidine analogue, was found to have caused the disease in a small group of drug addicts in the 1980s. No other environmental toxins are recognized.

Parkinson plus syndromes

A small proportion of patients who present with typical Parkinsonian symptoms turn out subsequently to have one of the Parkinson plus syndromes:

Progressive supranuclear palsy shows in addition a vertical supranuclear gaze palsy (downward movements before upward), axial rigidity and progressive dementia.

Multiple system atrophy shows in addition varying combinations of pyramidal (brisk reflexes, extensor plantar responses), cerebellar (dysarthria, ataxia) and autonomic (incontinence, postural hypotension) features.

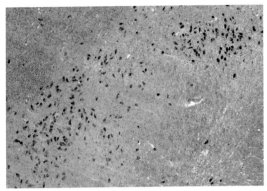

Fig. 99 Normal substantia nigra. Note normal complement of pigmented dopamine cells.

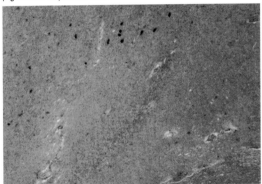

Fig. 100 Parkinsonian substantia nigra. Shows marked absence of pigmented cells.

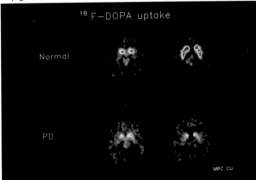

Fig. 101 A positron-emission tomograph showing reduced ¹⁸F-dopa uptake in the basal ganglia in Parkinson's disease (PD) compared to a normal subject.

Other basal ganglia disorders

Disease of the basal ganglia can lead to a variety of different movement abnormalities, such as chorea, athetosis, dystonia (Fig. 103) and ballismus. Very similar involuntary movements may occur due to a variety of different aetiologies. Wilson's disease, a defect of copper metabolism, must always be excluded since it is treatable.

Huntington's disease

This is a chronic degenerative disorder, particularly involving the caudate nucleus giving rise to chorea. It is inherited in an autosomal dominant pattern, and the abnormal gene has been located on chromosome 6. The DNA abnormality consists of a sequence of trinucleotide repeats, larger numbers of repeats being associated with earlier onset disease.

Clinical features

The main clinical features are choreiform movements and a progressive dementia, with an onset usually in the fourth or fifth decade. Initially, the chorea may be very mild, and may slowly develop with time. A positive family history is almost always available. The diagnosis is clinical and investigations are of little help.

Management

Treatment is unfortunately restricted to the chorea, when a dopamine receptor blocker such as tetrabenazine may be helpful. Prenatal identification of the abnormal gene is now possible, and families with cases of the disease require expert genetic counselling.

Other causes of chorea are Sydenham's chorea, associated with rheumatic fever in children, and neuroleptic drugs.

Athetosis

This is characterized by slow writhing postures of the limbs. It is mainly seen as a form of congenital cerebral palsy associated with anoxia, kernicterus or, in adults, following cerebral trauma.

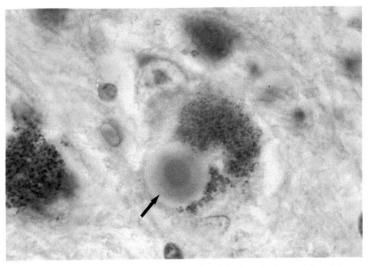

Fig. 102 Lewy body. High power photomicrographs of the Lewy body—an intracellular inclusion body.

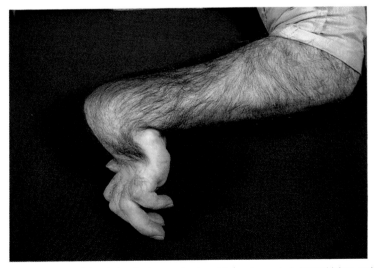

Fig. 103 A dystonic hand showing hyperextension at the metacarpal-phalangeal joints, and flexion at the wrist.

Dystonia

Dystonia is a movement disorder in which there are sustained muscle contractions, frequently causing twisting and repetitive movements, or abnormal postures (Fig. 103, p. 64). It may be localized or generalized.

Clinical features

When confined to one part of the body it is termed *focal*, when more of the body is affected it is termed *generalized dystonia*.

Adult onset *focal dystonias* occur 12 times more commonly than the generalized forms. The most common focal dystonias are blepharospasm (Fig. 104), spasmodic torticollis (Fig. 105) and occupational cramps, such as writer's cramp. Their onset is usually slowly progressive between the ages of 20 and 50 years, and affects both sexes.

Generalized dystonia occurs sporadically in a third of patients, and as an autosomal recessive or dominant in a further third. The remainder develop dystonia secondary to other disease, the most common being cerebral palsy and neuroleptic drugs. It may also occur in Wilson's disease. In *dystonia musculorum deformans* the onset is usually localized, starting before the age of 11 years and gradually becoming widespread.

Management

In general, treatment of these involuntary movements is unsatisfactory. Acute drug-induced dyskinesias should be treated with an intravenous anticholinergic such as procyclidine. Dystonia may be helped by high-dose anticholinergics or levodopa, and blepharospasm and spasmodic torticollis are treated symptomatically by injection of botulinum toxin into the orbicularis and neck muscles respectively.

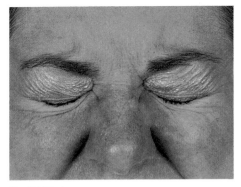

Fig. 104 Blepharospasm.

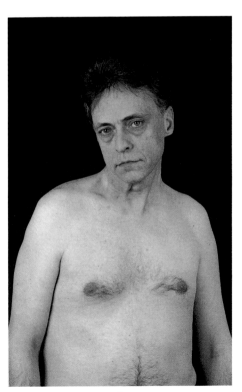

Fig. 105 Spasmodic torticollis.

In polyneuropathies, the peripheral nervous system is involved in a generalized disorder, either genetic, e.g. hereditary motor and sensory neuropathy (HMSN), or acquired, e.g. Guillain–Barré syndrome or diabetic neuropathy. In mononeuropathies, individual peripheral nerves or nerve roots are affected by local processes, such as pressure, entrapment, trauma, or inflammation.

Polyneuropathies

Clinical features

Polyneuropathies, e.g. HMSN (Charcot–Marie–Tooth syndrome), cause symmetrical distal sensory loss and distal weakness and wasting. Distal motor signs, e.g. wasting and weakness of the feet and legs (Fig. 106), are prominent in axonal neuropathies. In demyelinating neuropathies there is diffuse or even proximal weakness, with preserved muscle bulk and prominent dysaesthesiae or even pain. In some inherited progressive neuropathies, e.g. Refsum's disease and HMSN, there is maldevelopment of the distal parts of the limbs, especially the toes as with pes cavus (Fig. 107). In chronic demyelinating neuropathies and leprosy (Hansen's disease), there is hypertrophy of the cutaneous nerves (Fig. 108).

In long-standing peripheral neuropathies associated with severe distal sensory loss there is trophic damage to the tendons and joints leading to progressive deformity of the joints of the feet, ankles (Fig. 109, p. 70) and knees (Charcot joint deformities). ➡

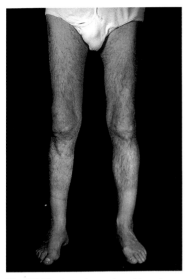

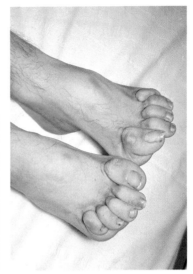

Fig. 106 Distal wasting and weakness in an axonal neuropathy.

Fig. 107 Pes cavus.

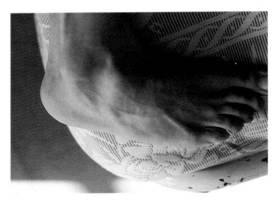

Fig. 108 Hypertrophy of the distal cutaneous branch of the sural nerve on the lateral border of the foot in HMSN type 1, a demyelinating neuropathy.

Look for signs of systemic disease, e.g. cancer, vasculitis, dysproteinaemia, leprosy and diabetes mellitus. Is there a family history? Is the neuropathy acute? Is there symmetrical polyneuropathy, mononeuropathy or multiple involvement of single nerves? Is there biochemical or imaging evidence of systemic disease? Is the motor or sensory conduction velocity slowed (<35 m/s) as in demyelinating neuropathy or is it more or less normal, as in axonal neuropathy? Is there conduction block, i.e. lower amplitude muscle action potential from proximal stimulation than from distal stimulation of the same nerve?

Nerve biopsy

The sural nerve near the ankle is usually used for biopsy because it is a pure sensory nerve that has only a small sensory representation on the skin. In chronic demyelinating neuropathies there is hyperplasia of Schwann cells, producing whorls of Schwann cell cytoplasm which resemble onion bulbs, interspersed with fibrous tissue (Fig. 110). In axonal neuropathies there is 'dying back' of the distal parts of the axons, with secondary loss of myelin from these distal portions of the damaged axons. ➡

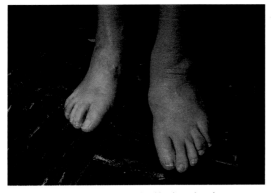

Fig. 109 Deformity of the toes and ankles in a chronic neuropathy.

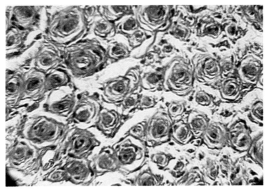

Fig. 110 Onion-bulb hyperplasia of Schwann cells in a chronic demyelinating neuropathy.

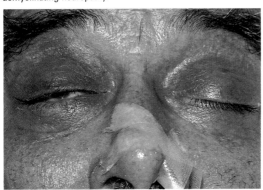

Fig. 111 Bilateral facial weakness in Guillain–Barré neuropathy.

Guillain–Barré syndrome

This is an acute inflammatory demyelinating polyneuropathy that usually follows a minor acute infection. There is distal and/or proximal weakness, often affecting the face (Fig. 111, p. 70), with frequent involvement of respiratory muscles and some distal sensory loss. The reflexes are usually lost. Assess ventilatory capacity carefully. Although the prognosis for recovery is excellent, treatment with IV gamma globulin or plasma exchange is often used at presentation. A rare relapsing and chronic form of the disorder is steroid-responsive. Cases following *C. jejuni* infection are especially severe and may be primarily axonal.

Other polyneuropathies

Hansen's disease (leprosy): can cause *ulnar nerve palsy* (Fig. 112), which leads to weakness of all intrinsic muscles, with a characteristic posture of interphalangeal flexion and metacarpophalangeal extension, affecting the medial two digits. Hypo-esthetic, depigmented skin lesions and nodular enlargement of peripheral nerves, especially cutaneous nerves occur.

Hereditary amyloid neuropathies: amyloid (Fig. 113) is deposited in peripheral nerves, causing hypertrophied nerves with damage to the myelin sheath of affected nerve fibres, and therefore slowed nerve conduction velocity.

Paraproteinaemia: can also cause neuropathy, and nerve biopsy may show deposition of IgM protein in relation to myelin sheaths (Fig. 114).

Charcot–Marie–Tooth disease (HMSN): a group of hereditary neuropathies with several different clinical types and genetic loci. The Type 1 disorder is demyelinating and the Type 2 is axonal in type. Hereditary liability to pressure palsies is a disorder related to Type 1 HMSN due to a point mutation or deletion at the same locus.

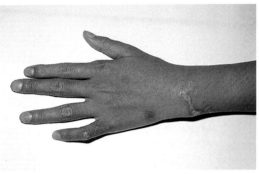

Fig. 112 Ulnar nerve palsy, with typical finger deformity.

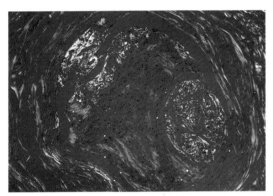

Fig. 113 Apple-green fluorescence of amyloid deposition seen in a nerve biopsy stained with Congo red.

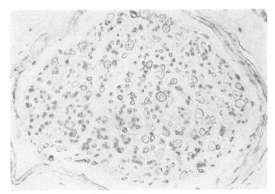

Fig. 114 Brown staining with immunoperoxidase representing IgM deposition in neuropathy associated with IgM paraproteinaemia.

Mononeuropathies

Aetiology

The median, ulnar, radial and common peroneal nerves, and the lateral cutaneous nerve of the thigh are commonly damaged by external pressure, direct injury or by entrapment in interosseous and ligamentous canals.

Clinical types

Median nerve palsy: (Fig. 115) most often caused by entrapment in the carpal tunnel on the flexor aspect of the wrist. The nerve is trapped and compressed at this site, resulting in weakness and wasting of the thenar eminence, with sensory disturbance in the median-innervated skin of the hand. There is pain in the hand and also often the forearm, especially at night. EMG studies show slowed nerve conduction velocity across the carpal tunnel.

Ulnar nerve palsy: atrophy and weakness of intrinsic hand muscles (Fig. 116), with sensory loss on the medial border of the hand. The nerve is usually damaged by pressure at the elbow (in the olecranon groove), and there is tenderness at this site with pain referred into the distribution of the nerve in the hand. There is a typical deformity of the medial two digits (Fig. 112).

Radial nerve palsy: usually due to pressure injury in the spiral groove of the humerus or fracture of the humerus. It presents with wrist and finger drop.

Common peroneal nerve palsy: presents with weakness of ankle dorsiflexion and eversion, and sensory impairment on the lateral aspect of the foot and leg. The ankle jerk is normal.

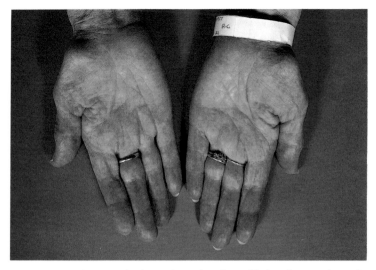

Fig. 115 Bilateral thenar wasting in carpal tunnel syndrome. The hypothenar eminence is normal.

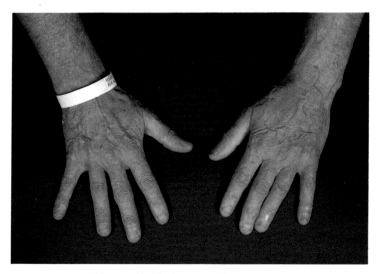

Fig. 116 Weakness of interossei in left ulnar nerve palsy.

Duchenne muscular dystrophy

This X-linked myopathy is a severe progressive disorder, affecting 1 in 3500 male births. The disorder progresses from difficulty walking and climbing at age 3–5 years, to total dependency by about the age of 12 years and death around the age of 20 years.

Aetiology

The disorder is associated with absence of dystrophin, a constituent of the cytoskeletal framework of the muscle cell membrane. The gene encoding dystrophin is located on the short arm of the X chromosome at the Xp21 position, the site of a deletion responsible for most cases of the disease. Absence of this gene can be recognized in white blood cells. *Becker's muscular dystrophy* is a less severe form of the Xp21 disorder, presenting in older boys with a slower progression.

Clinical features

Cardiac involvement is frequent, but the external ocular, pelvic sphincter and distal hand muscles tend to be spared. Affected limb muscles, especially calves and deltoids, usually show hypertrophy from fibrosis and fatty infiltration in the earlier stages (Fig. 117). Joint contractures and respiratory difficulties develop.

Investigations

The *muscle biopsy* (Fig. 118) shows increased thickness of interfascicular and endomysial fibrous connective tissue (blue-green in illustration), large rounded, densely stained 'hyaline' fibres and smaller rounded fibres, with foci of degeneration and regeneration of individual fibres.

CT scans of limb and girdle muscles are valuable in the assessment of muscle disease (Fig. 119). In this example of Becker's disease, there is marked involvement of the flexor muscles of the thigh, with less severe involvement of the anterior thigh and gracilis muscles.

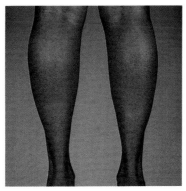

Fig. 117 Hypertrophy of calves in Duchenne muscular dystrophy.

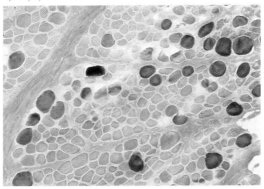

Fig. 118 Muscle biopsy in Duchenne dystrophy.

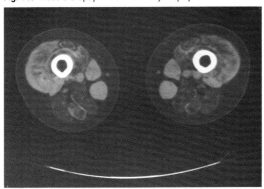

Fig. 119 Involvement of thigh muscles in a case of Becker's dystrophy. The low attenuation flexor muscles are severely involved.

Facioscapulohumeral muscular dystrophy

This is an uncommon dominantly inherited disease that is a specific clinical syndrome, but with several different causes, classified separately from the larger group of limb-girdle dystrophies by its characteristic features.

Clinical features

Weakness particularly affects face, periscapular muscles and biceps brachii with similar involvement of thigh and pelvic girdle muscles in the later stages of the disease (Fig. 120). Life expectancy is only relatively unaffected.

Oculopharyngeal muscular dystrophy

This condition involves ocular and pharyngeal muscles (Fig. 121). Pure ocular myopathy also occurs as a dominantly inherited disorder.

Clinical features

There is ptosis and paralysis of the external ocular muscles, without involvement of the internal ocular muscles.

Scapuloperoneal muscular dystrophy

Periscapular muscles are relatively selectively affected in scapuloperoneal muscular dystrophy (Fig. 122).

Clinical features

Weakness of the periscapular muscles makes the shoulders unstable, because of the inability to fix the position of the scapulae against a load.

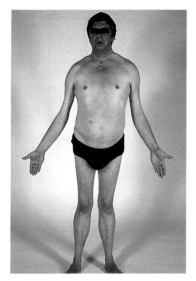

Fig. 120 Facioscapulohumeral muscular dystrophy, showing atrophy of proximal and upper arm muscles, with lordosis and facial involvement.

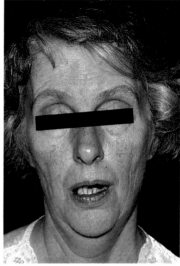

Fig. 121 Oculopharyngeal muscular dystrophy, with ptosis, weakness of extraocular muscles and facial and bulbar muscular weakness.

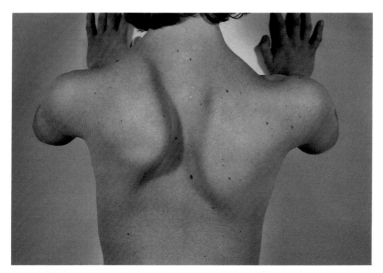

Fig. 122 Weakness of periscapular muscles causes winging of the scapulae.

Myotonic dystrophy

Clinical features

This is a dominantly inherited disorder. Myotonia consists of a persistent contraction of muscle fibres following cessation of voluntary contraction or after a mechanical stimulus. In myotonic dystrophy there is myotonia, with ptosis and weakness of the face, the distal limb muscles and the sternomastoids. This produces a characteristic facial and bodily appearance, with a wasted neck and face (Figs 123 & 124). Cardiomyopathy with arrhythmias, oesophageal dysfunction, constipation, mild glucose intolerance and testicular atrophy are frequent features. Patients with myotonic dystrophy are often poorly adjusted socially. In other separately inherited *congenital myotonic syndromes*, myotonia occurs without dystrophic features.

Investigations

The EMG is diagnostic; the myotonic discharges produce a 'dive-bomber' sound of varying frequency and amplitude that can be recorded as a series of spike discharges (Fig. 125). The genetic locus on chromosome 19 is defined and consists of a sequence of trinucleotide repeats, accounting for the variable age of onset and severity of the disorder.

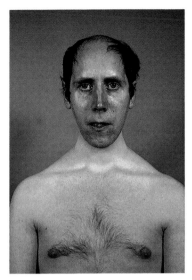

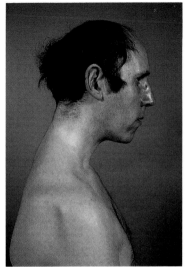

Fig. 123 Myotonic dystrophy, showing frontal baldness and characteristic facial appearance.

Fig. 124 Weakness of sternomastoids and neck extensors is a feature of myotonic dystrophy.

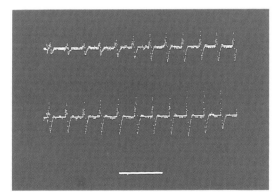

Fig. 125 Myotonic discharges on an EMG, showing the incremental amplitude and gradually changing frequency of the discharge from a single muscle fibre. Bar: 20 ms.

Inflammatory myopathies

Dermatomyositis and polymyositis

These are common, acquired myopathies characterized by autoimmune-mediated muscle fibre necrosis. Dermatomyositis is usually acute, and in adults (usually older than 50 years) may be a manifestation of cancer. The childhood variety of the disease has a marked vascular component. Polymyositis also occurs as a component of mixed connective tissue disease. There is muscle tenderness, weakness and, in dermatomyositis, a violaceous rash, especially in areas exposed to light. The ESR and creatine kinase are raised, and the EMG and muscle biopsy are diagnostic (Fig. 126).

Metabolic myopathies

These include glycogen storage diseases, mitochondrial myopathies, periodic paralyses and malignant hyperpyrexia. These are inherited disorders of metabolism, often but not necessarily restricted to muscle, usually due to single enzyme deficiencies. Acid maltase deficiency is a late onset progressive myopathy, causing weakness, fatigue and diaphragmatic paralysis leading to sleep apnoea. The vacuolar appearance of the muscle biopsy is due to accumulation of glycogen within lysosomes (Fig. 127).

Mitochondrial myopathies

In mitochondrial myopathies, fatigue and lactic acidosis are the main features. There are accumulations of abnormal, enlarged mitochondria at the edges of type 1 muscle fibres, shown in the NADH reaction (Fig. 128). Renal tubular acidosis and CNS involvement occur in some cases. The mitochondrial myoencephalopathies are maternally inherited and mostly due to defects in mitochondrial DNA.

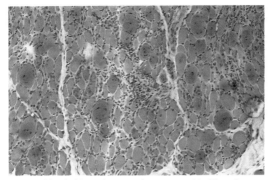

Fig. 126 Muscle biopsy in acute dermatomyositis. There is a diffuse inflammatory cell response, with muscle fibre necrosis and regeneration.

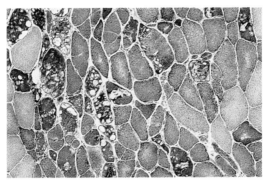

Fig. 127 Acid maltase deficiency (adult-onset type). There is a prominent vacuolar myopathy.

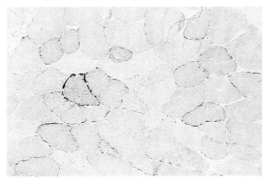

Fig. 128 Mitochondrial myopathy showing accumulation of mitochondria at the edges of type 1 muscle fibres as succinic dehydrogenase-positive structures.

Myasthenia gravis is an autoimmune disease in which an IgG antibody is directed against a component of the acetylcholine receptor antigen complex at the post-synaptic part of the neuromuscular junction. These receptors are nicotinic cholinergic receptors. There is an association with autoimmune thyroid disease.

Clinical features

There is fluctuating weakness and fatiguability during exercise, worse at the end of the day and relieved by rest. Ptosis (Fig. 129) and weakness of external ocular muscles (Fig. 130) are common; diplopia is the presenting feature in 40% of cases. The ocular muscles often show apparent bilateral lateral rectus weakness. Distal hand muscles are next most commonly affected, and the disease reaches its maximal severity about a year after the onset. This and weakness of other muscles worsens with repeated movement or maintenance of a posture. There is no sensory loss and the tendon reflexes are normal.

Investigations

EMG shows a characteristic decrement in the amplitude of the muscle action potential evoked by a supramaximal electrical stimulus to the nerve supplying the muscle tested (Fig. 131). In health, the fourth potential of a sequence elicited at 2–3 Hz should not be less than 10% smaller than the first. ➡

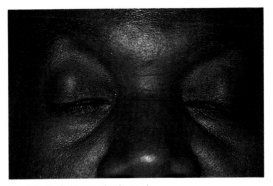

Fig. 129 Ptosis in myasthenia gravis.

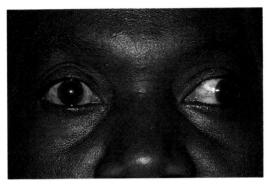

Fig. 130 Same patient in Figure 129 after intravenous edrophonium (with improvement in ptosis) to show weakness of extraocular muscles.

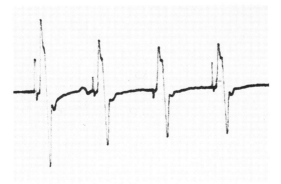

Fig. 131 Decrement in amplitude of evoked muscle action potential in 2 Hz train of stimuli to the motor nerve.

Management

The response to anticholinesterase treatment, e.g. pyridostigmine, neostigmine, is both dramatic and diagnostic, but treatment consists not only of anticholinesterase drugs, but of immunosuppression with azathoprine or, in severe cases, with gradually incrementing oral steroid. Plasma exchange is also used to remove circulating antibody.

Thymectomy is used to induce remission, especially in the first 2 years of the disease. It is indicated at the time of diagnosis in all patients, except in the very old and those with mild ocular symptoms. In about half of men with myasthenia, and in about 10% of patients overall, there is a thymoma, a benign tumour that can usually be detected by radiography or CT scanning of the chest (Fig. 132). In other patients, hyperplasia of the thymus is found (Fig. 133). This thymic abnormality is important in initiating the disturbed immune response that causes the defect in neuromuscular transmission.

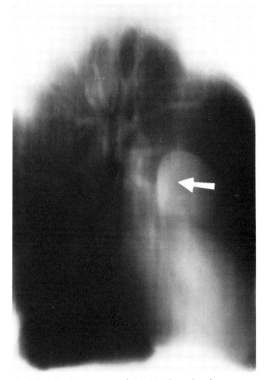

Fig. 132 Lateral tomogram of chest to show thymic enlargement. The mass is a rounded opacity lying just above and anterior to the heart (arrow).

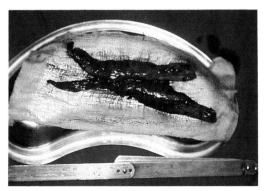

Fig. 133 Thymic enlargement in specimen removed from patient with myasthenia gravis.

Motor neuron disease (amyotrophic lateral sclerosis) is an acquired degenerative disorder of the lower and upper motor neurons.

Clinical features

The disorder causes progressive weakness, usually asymmetrical at the onset, with wasting, fasciculation, and spasticity and extensor plantar responses. Life expectancy is about 1–5 years. There are no sensory abnormalities, and the external ocular and sphincter muscles are not involved until the terminal stages. The intrinsic hand muscles are often involved early (Figs 134 & 135), and there is usually wasting and fasciculation of the tongue (Fig. 136). Presentation with bulbar palsy, causing difficulty speaking and swallowing, and later weakness of ventilatory muscles carries a poor prognosis. Fasciculation often affects muscles that have not yet begun to show atrophy. A few cases are familial.

Differential diagnosis

The diagnosis depends on recognition of the characteristic features, and exclusion of other disorders, especially cervical spondylosis with myelopathy, and chronic motor neuropathy (multifocal motor neuropathy) in which fasciculation may occur.

Some hereditary cases have been associated with abnormalities in the Cu-Zn superoxide dysmutase gene on chromosome 21, suggesting an excitotoxic aetiology for this form of the disease. ➡

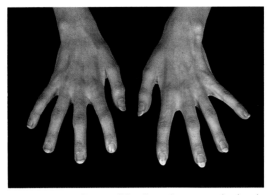

Fig. 134 Wasting of the small hand muscles seen on the dorsal surfaces in motor neuron disease.

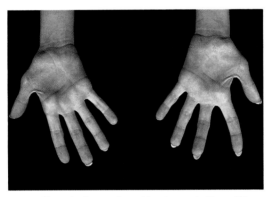

Fig. 135 View of palmar surface of hands seen in Figure 134.

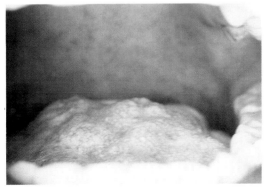

Fig. 136 Wasting of the tongue (which was also fasciculating).

The EMG shows chronic partial denervation with fasciculations and fibrillations, and normal motor and sensory conduction.

Since there is loss of anterior horn cells and of motor cells in the somatic motor nuclei in the brainstem, neurogenic atrophy of muscle develops. This is accompanied by reinnervation by nearby, relatively healthy motor neurons through axonal sprouting. Normal skeletal muscle contains a pseudomosaic of muscle fibres of the three main histochemical types (types 1, 2a and 2b fibres) in an approximately equal quantity (Fig. 137). In motor neuron disease, reinnervation is fairly effective in the early stages, and about 30% of motor neurons are lost before atrophy occurs. In atrophic muscles there is fibre type grouping in which clusters of fibres of the same histochemical type are found, resulting from axonal sprouting and reinnervation of nearby denervated fibres (Fig. 138).

The second illustration shows rather rounded fibres, with fibre type grouping and groups of atrophic denervated fibres. This was seen in a patient with type 3 spinal muscular atrophy, an autosomal recessive disorder in which anterior horn cells degenerate during a period of several decades, but in which there are no upper motor neuron features.

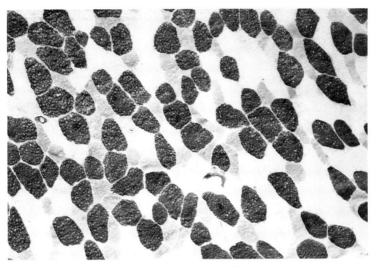

Fig. 137 Pseudomosaic distribution of type 1, 2a and 2b fibres in normal muscle.

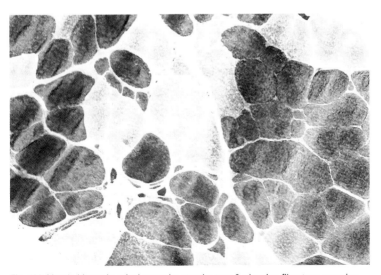

Fig. 138 Muscle biopsy in spinal muscular atrophy type 3, showing fibre type grouping with a cluster of atrophic denervated muscle fibres. There is hypertrophy of many of the reinnervated muscle fibres.

27 / Spinal cord disease

Aetiology

Degenerative disease: causes can be grouped under two types:
- *of the vertebral column*: cervical spondylosis (Fig. 139), rheumatoid arthritis and calcification of the posterior longitudinal ligament.
- *of the spinal cord*: subacute combined degeneration of the cord (B_{12} deficiency), Friedreich's ataxia, hereditary spastic paraparesis and motor neuron disease.

Neoplastic: extradural metastasis, intradural meningioma or neurofibroma, intramedullary astrocytoma or ependymoma, paraneoplastic syndrome.

Infective: poliomyelitis, herpes zoster virus, post-infectious/vaccination, tropical spastic paraparesis (HTLV-1), AIDS (HIV), syphilis (usually tabes dorsalis), Lyme disease (borreliosis) and tuberculosis (usually extradural abscess).

Developmental: syringomyelia (Fig. 140).

Vascular: arteriovenous malformations (Figs 141 & 142) and spinal cord infarction.

Demyelinating: multiple sclerosis, radiotherapy and chemotherapy.

Traumatic: spinal cord injury.

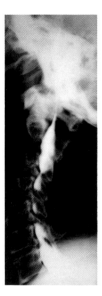

Fig. 139 Spinal cord compression in cervical spondylosis with osteophytes indenting the theca anteriorly and ligamentous buckling posteriorly.

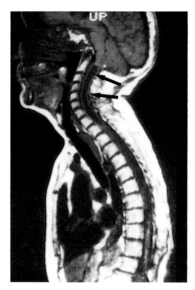

Fig. 140 Syringomyelia (arrows) in brain and spinal cord MRI, in this case, associated with Paget's disease.

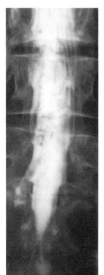

Fig. 141 Spinal angioma. Myelography shows filling defects due to large serpiginous draining veins.

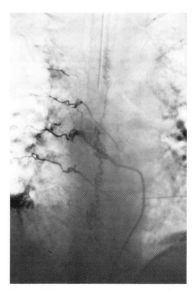

Fig. 142 Spinal arteriography showing dural AVM in upper thoracic region with large draining veins above and below.

Approach

To plan the investigative tests appropriately, analyse the sequence of symptoms and signs.

Decide whether the lesion is more likely to be either:

- *intrinsic*: sphincter disturbance, segmental pain and temperature loss with spontaneous pain, loss of jerks, segmental wasting and weakness, paraparesis and posterior column loss
- *extrinsic* (compression): radicular features, paraparesis (often asymmetric or of the Brown–Séquard type), rising sensory level and sphincter disturbance.

Determine the upper level at the bedside, remembering that clinical levels are often suspended well below the actual level of the responsible lesion.

Clinical tests and investigations

Blood tests include WR, B_{12} and virus studies if indicated. X-rays are indicated for narrow canal or pathological widening, disc disease, atlanto-axial subluxation, bony deposits and tuberculosis. Full length myelography, MRI or CT (Figs 143–146) pick up most compressive causes and syringomyelia, and where available MR imaging has replaced CT myelography. CSF may be helpful with infective causes and demyelination (MR imaging is sensitive here). Others tests include spinal angiography (if large draining veins are seen on myelography), EMG in suspected motor neuron disease and, occasionally, bone scans. Often a diagnosis is only made at operative decompression.

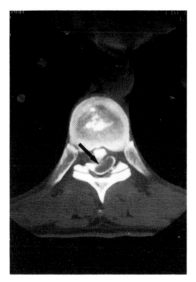

Fig. 143 Calcified degenerate thoracic disc compressing spinal cord (arrow) seen on CT myelogram.

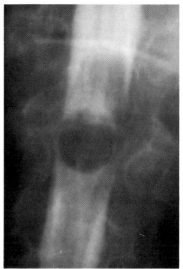

Fig. 144 Myelography showing an intradural mass lesion.

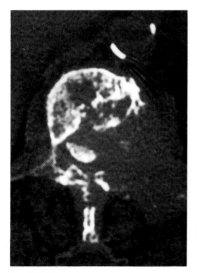

Fig. 145 CT myelogram showing extensive extradural spinal metastatic disease.

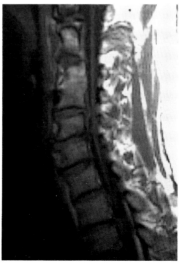

Fig. 146 MRI cervical spine, showing prolapsed C3/4 disc compressing the cord.

28 / Radiculopathy

Aetiology

Conditions often associated with radiculopathy include:
- spondylosis and osteophyte formation
- prolapse of degenerate disc material
- bony metastasis or infections
- trauma
- cervical ribs (Fig. 147)
- neurofibromas (Figs 148 & 149)
- herpes zoster virus infections
- neuralgic amyotrophy.

Clinical features

Symptoms include shooting pains, paraesthesias and numbness, often associated with neck stiffness or low back pain. Symptoms often worsen during sneezing, coughing and straining, and during movement and exercise. Signs to look for include limited movements of the neck or lumbosacral spine, with impaired straight leg raising. Muscle weakness, loss of reflexes and sensory impairment occur in appropriate myotomal and dermatomal distributions. The most common radiculopathies are C6 and C7 in the upper limb, and L5 and S1 in the legs.

Investigations

Plain X-rays can be used to detect narrowing of disc spaces. Good oblique views should be obtained to visualize the intervertebral root exit foramina (Fig. 148).

The current definitive investigation involves CT either alone or more usually combined with myelography (Figs 150, 151 & 152, p. 98) or MR imaging.

Nerve conduction studies are helpful in excluding a peripheral nerve lesion, and EMG is helpful in confirming evidence of denervation in a radicular distribution, and defines the limits of the radicular involvement. ➡

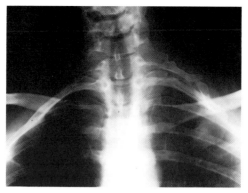

Fig. 147 Left cervical rib.

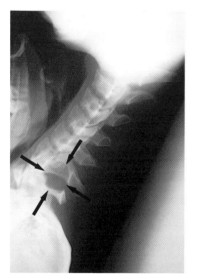

Fig. 148 Expansion of C2 intervertebral foramen due to neurofibroma (arrow).

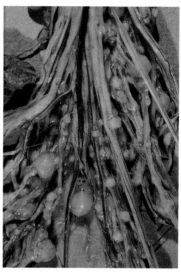

Fig. 149 Multiple neurofibromas on the cauda equina at post-mortem.

All radiculopathies should be managed conservatively in the initial stage. Non-steroidal anti-inflammatory drugs should be tried in ali cases. Traction may be used. The neck should be immobilized using a combination of hard and soft collars. The back should be rested in bed with a firm mattress. Once the symptoms have abated, carefully graded exercises with progressive mobilization should ensure continuing clinical improvement. Swimming is an excellent way of building up paravertebral muscle strength. Surgery should be considered if the symptoms, particularly pain, do not respond to medical treatment, or if there is progressive muscle weakness.

Lumbar canal stenosis

This is a further cause of lumbosacral radiculopathies, and occurs most often in association with a congenitally narrow spinal canal (Fig. 153). Patients complain of lower limb cramps and aches on standing and walking and often there is numbness and weakness of the legs as well. Low back pain is variable and sphincter disturbance distinctly uncommon. Typically these symptoms remit with rest and by extending the spine and flexing the legs at hip and knee joints. Decompression of the lumbar canal at multiple levels is usually required.

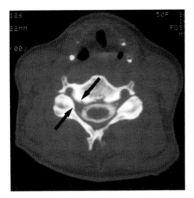

Fig. 150 CT myelogram showing right osteophytic encroachment. Compare diameter of exit foramina (arrows) on the two sides.

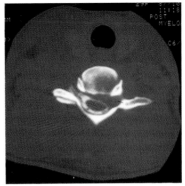

Fig. 151 CT myelogram showing cervical disc prolapse on left, compressing exiting root and displacing spinal cord.

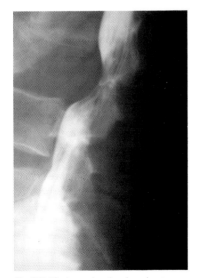

Fig. 152 Myelography showing ghost lumbar vertebral body due to bony metastasis and complicating cauda equina compression.

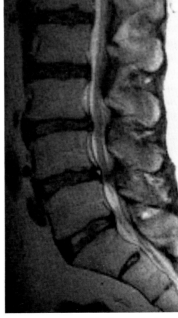

Fig. 153 MR image of lumbosacral spine showing hour-glass deformity of the spinal canal due to canal stenosis.

Hydrocephalus

This is the most common developmental abnormality, either as a primary abnormality or as a feature of other defects of development of the neural tube, e.g. in dysraphisms such as spina bifida, or in Arnold–Chiari malformation.

Aetiology

In infancy, hydrocephalus (Fig. 154) is usually due to obstruction of flow of CSF, often in the aqueduct of Sylvius. This causes CSF to accumulate in the lateral and third ventricles, causing dilatation of these ventricles (Fig. 155) and raised intracranial pressure.

Clinical features

The disorder may develop very slowly, presenting with increasing size of the head and ocular signs, especially resting-downward deviation with slight dilatation of the pupils. There may be developmental retardation with floppy tone. Ventricular dilatation causes narrowing of the white matter of the brain, but no abnormality of the grey matter. Papilloedema may occur.

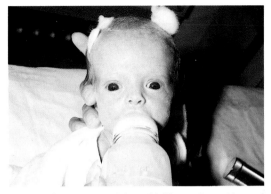

Fig. 154 Infantile hydrocephalus, with lid retraction and 'sunset' eye position.

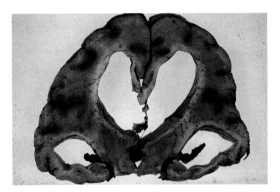

Fig. 155 Dilatation of lateral and third ventricles in hydrocephalus due to aqueductal stenosis.

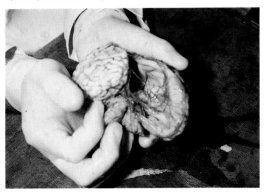

Fig. 156 Failure of normal development of the corpus callosum.

Other developmental abnormalities

Other developmental abnormalities involve the brain itself, e.g. agenesis of the corpus callosum (Fig. 156, p. 100), sometimes causing complex psychometric defects, porencephaly (probably due to infarction in a vascular territory) and failure of migration of cells, resulting in cortical dysplasias that may lead to epilepsy. Craniofacial malformations are often not accompanied by brain malformations.

Hemiatrophy of the brain

Hemiatrophy of the brain is clinically important because it is found in people with hemiparesis, smallness of the affected limbs, focal and generalized seizures and (sometimes) intellectual retardation. The hemisphere opposite the abnormal limbs is atrophic (Fig. 157) probably because of infarction sustained in utero or in the perinatal period (Davidoff–Dyke malformation).

Cerebellar atrophy

This may occur as a primary malformation, or may develop as part of a progressive degeneration of the cerebellum and its connexions (Fig. 158). This group of disorders is classified according to genetic or biochemical causation (when this is known), or according to its associated clinical features, e.g. olivopontinocerebellar degeneration or pure cerebellar degeneration. Cerebellar atrophy also occurs after poisoning with certain drugs, especially phenytoin, and in alcoholics.

Arnold–Chiari malformation

In this malformation there is elongation of the cerebellar vermis, with herniation of this tissue and of the cerebellar tonsils and medulla downward into the foramen magnum (Fig. 159). Obstruction of the outlets of the fourth ventricle may result in hydrocephalus. This malformation is often associated with lumbosacral spina bifida. ➡

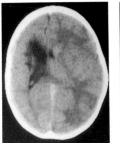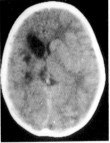

Fig. 157 Hemiatrophy of the right hemisphere, with a porencephalic cystic cavity in the frontal white matter. Contiguous axial slices seen on cerebral CT.

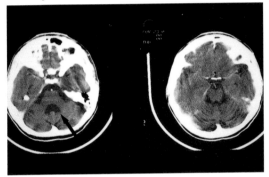

Fig. 158 Cerebellar atrophy. Axial views at the level of the pons (left) and the midbrain (right). Note prominent cerebellar folia and enlargement of the fourth ventricle (arrow).

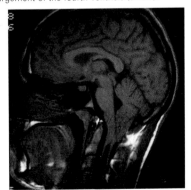

Fig. 159 Chiari malformation (MRI scan). The lower brainstem is enlongated, and the tonsils lie in the upper spinal canal below the plane of the foramen magnum.

Neurofibromatosis

Type 1 neurofibromatosis (NF1; von Recklinghausen's disease) is an inherited neurocutaneous syndrome (Fig. 160) in which multiple *café au lait* spots, freckling, and cutaneous nodules consisting of hard and soft (plexiform) neuromas occur. Peripheral nerves may be nodular with neurofibromas, and there is a propensity to develop CNS tumours, especially neurofibromas, meningiomas and gliomas, and tumours of other organs, e.g. phaeochromocytomas. The latter may present with hypertension. Mental retardation and macrocephaly may occur. The gene for the disorder is encoded on chromosome 17, and genetic counselling is possible by linkage markers in families with two or more affected members.

The Type 2 disorder (NF2) consists of bilateral acoustic neuromas with few if any cutaneous stigmata of the disease. This related syndrome is due to a different chromosomal abnormality.

Incontinentia pigmenti

This presents with red lesions (Fig. 161) that become pigmented within 3 months of birth. There may be associated mental retardation and patent ductus arteriosus.

Osler–Rendu–Weber syndrome

This is an inherited form of capillary malformation in which there are widespread vascular malformations, involving skin (Fig. 162) lungs, liver, and mucous membranes. The CNS is only rarely involved.

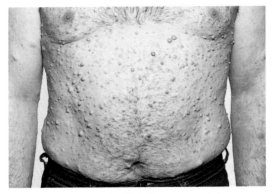

Fig. 160 Neurofibromatosis (NF1). The cutaneous lesions are characteristic.

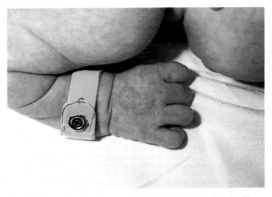

Fig. 161 Incontinentia pigmenti. The lesions on the hand will later become pigmented.

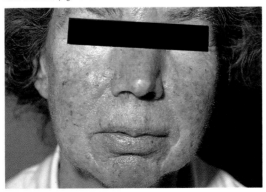

Fig. 162 Osler–Rendu–Weber syndrome.

Head injuries are a common cause of disability. In *closed* head injuries there is no penetration of the brain's coverings. In *open* head injury the brain is exposed, or penetrated, allowing the possibility of direct injury and infection. Most head injuries are closed. These result in *concussion* or *contusion*, or even in *haemorrhage* into the brain or into the subdural or extradural spaces. Always exclude an associated injury of the cervical spine.

Concussion

Simple concussion is due to sudden accelerative forces applied to the brain, causing transient distortion of the brain within the cranial cavity. There may be axonal injury, particularly caused by physical disruption of axons (Fig. 163).

Clinical features

The clinical features depend on the forces involved; the severity of the injury can be estimated from the duration of the post-traumatic amnesia.

Contusion

Cerebral contusion (Fig. 164) occurs from haemorrhage into the brain, usually *contre coup* to the site of the injury and most often in the frontal, temporal or occipital regions, at the white matter/grey matter junction (Fig. 165).

Clinical features

It is nearly always associated with severe concussive brain injury, and carries a higher risk of residual cerebral deficit and of post-traumatic epilepsy. In fatal cases of closed head injury there is a combination of cerebral white matter oedema (due to widespread, severe axonal disruption) and contusion.

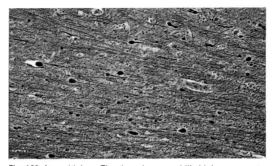

Fig. 163 Axonal injury. The densely agyrophilic blobs represent extruded axoplasmic material from severed axons, and associated glial reaction.

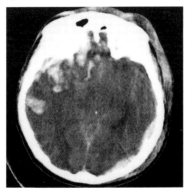

Fig. 164 Frontotemporal contusions shown by focal zones of increased density in subcortical parts of right side of the brain.

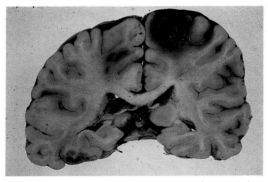

Fig. 165 This brain is swollen, with obliteration of the sulci of both hemispheres. There are subcortical haemorrhagic contusions, especially in the left parafalcine region.

Haemorrhage

Subdural haematoma (Fig. 166) consists of bleeding in the subdural potential space, usually from a ruptured vein.

Clinical features

There may be a delay of hours, days or even weeks before presentation with gradual impairment of consciousness or progressive loss of focal functions, e.g. hemiparesis. The haematoma consists of a collection of old and new haemorrhage of variable attenuation on CT scanning. There is often marked lateral shift of the brain with compression of the lateral ventricles, and transtentorial herniation (Fig. 167). The latter results in secondary impairment of brainstem function, with ipsilateral third nerve palsy (dilatation of the pupil followed by ptosis and extra-ocular muscle weakness) and compression of the contralateral pyramid against the tentorial edge. Later, unless the haematoma is removed, the ponto-mesencephalic respiratory centres are depressed and death results. The medial temporal lobe is herniated downward through the tentorial notch (Fig. 167), directly compressing the brainstem (uncal herniation).

A skull fracture (Fig. 168) increases the chance of the development of intracranial bleeding. If there is a displacement of the fracture into the brain (depressed fracture), this may need surgical debridement. Cortical injury increases the probability of the later development of epilepsy.

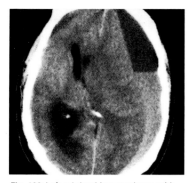

Fig. 166 Left subdural haemorrhage, with variable density in the haematoma, and obstruction and enlargement of the contralateral ventricle. There is displacement of the left hemisphere across the midline.

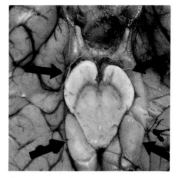

Fig. 167 Uncal herniation through the tentorium. The uncus of both temporal lobes has been squeezed downward through the tentorial notch (arrows), causing compression of the brain stem.

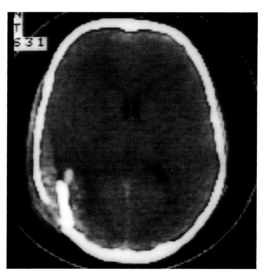

Fig. 168 Depressed skull fracture.

At post-mortem the brainstem shows haemorrhages in its rostral portion (Duret haemorrhages), as evidence of severe compression associated with massively increased intracranial pressure and death from brainstem compression (Fig. 170). The brain in this patient was oedematous and showed multiple contusions (Fig. 169).

Spinal injuries

The spine may also be injured in cases of head trauma. Most cervical injuries occur at C5/6, and may cause paraplegia or quadriplegia. It is important to consider the possibility of unstable cervical spine fracture in patients complaining of severe pain and stiffness of the neck after head injury. Atlanto-occipital subluxation, where the head is partially dislocated from the very top of the spinal column, is rare and always fatal (Fig. 171).

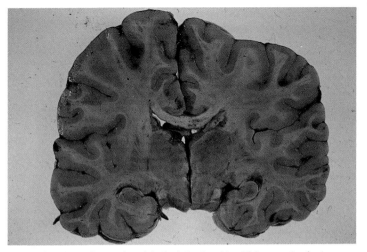

Fig. 169 Swelling and contusion of the brain in closed head injury causing fatal brainstem compression from transtentorial herniation.

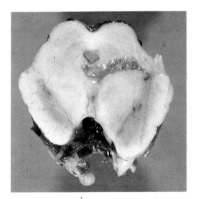

Fig. 170 Midbrain haemorrhages in fatal brainstem compression associated with head injury.

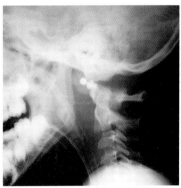

Fig. 171 Traumatic atlanto-occipital subluxation.

31 / Coma

Aetiology

Coma can result from a wide variety of structural and metabolic conditions. These include:
- haemorrhage, infarct, tumour, abscess
- closed head injury
- meningitis and encephalitis
- ictal and post-ictal states
- drug toxicity
- hypo- and hyperglycaemia
- hypo- and hyperthermia
- hypoxia
- hypopituitarism
- hypothyroidism
- Addison's disease
- hepatic (Fig. 172) or renal failure
- nutritional causes.

Clinical tests

It is important to assess the airway, breathing, circulation, level of consciousness, and brainstem function (pupils, eye movements and vestibulo-ocular reflexes, corneal, gag, coughing and swallowing reflexes, rate and rhythm of respiration). Check the neck for rigidity and the limbs for posture, tone, spontaneous movements, response to pain and reflexes.

Laboratory tests

These include tests for urea and electrolytes, blood sugar, calcium, liver function and blood gases. Consider drug screen, thyroid tests and cortisol. If no obvious cause is found, perform cranial CT (Fig. 173) or MRI, EEG (Fig. 174) and CSF examination.

Management

Ensure the patient is well oxygenated, give intravenous glucose and thiamine, control blood pressure and seizures, treat infections, correct acid-base disturbances and consider naloxone. In intracranial hypertension, give mannitol, steroids and ventilation.

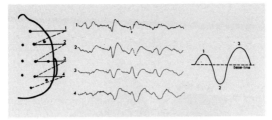

Fig. 172 Triphasic waves seen on EEG in coma resulting from liver failure.

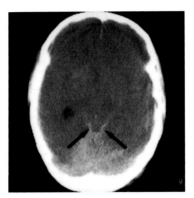

Fig. 173 CT brain scan showing generalized brain swelling with effacement of basal cisterns (arrows).

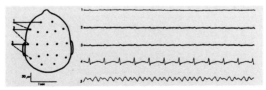

Fig. 174 Isoelectric EEG in comatose patient. ECG (channel 4) artefact is seen over the head. Channel 5 records respiratory movements.

Dementia is a condition resulting in a progressive impairment of cognitive function. Although this is usually global, in the early stages it may be selective.

Clinical features

These vary depending on the underlying aetiology but include impairment of memory (especially short-term), speech, calculations, writing, orientation and praxis.

Aetiology

When trying to establish the underlying aetiology in a patient with dementia, it is important to exclude treatable conditions (some 15% of the total) and to rule out psychiatric disorders (e.g. depression) which may mimic dementia.

The causes of dementia are:

- *Degenerative*: the most common cause of dementia over the age of 60 years is *Alzheimer's* disease. Its causation is still not understood, but it shows a typical pathological picture of cortical atrophy with senile plaques and neurofibrillary tangles (Figs 175 & 177). Other degenerative causes include Pick's disease, Huntington's chorea, multisystem atrophy and late Parkinson's disease.
- *Vascular*: multiple cerebral infarcts (Fig. 176) and diffuse small vessel disease.
- *Neoplastic*: frontal tumours and metastases.
- *Trauma*: chronic subdural haematoma.
- *Infection*: syphilis, Creutzfeldt–Jakob disease, AIDS-related dementia (Fig. 178) and subacute sclerosing panencephalitis (SSPE).
- *Toxic*: alcohol, lead and carbon monoxide.
- *Metabolic*: hypothyroidism and hepatic failure, uraemia, B_{12} deficiency, prolonged hypoglycaemia and prolonged hypoxia.
- *Psychiatric*: depression.

Management

Once the main treatable causes have been eliminated, management is largely supportive. Patients with dementia cause considerable strains on their immediate family and eventually institutional care is usually required.

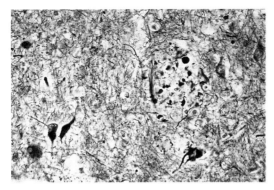

Fig. 175 Alzheimer's disease. A photomicrograph shows neurofibrillary tangles (right centre) and senile plaques (lower left).

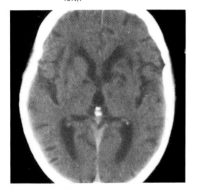

Fig. 176 Multiple infarct dementia.

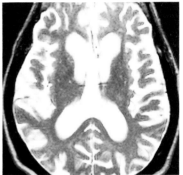

Fig. 177 Alzheimer's disease with marked cerebral atrophy.

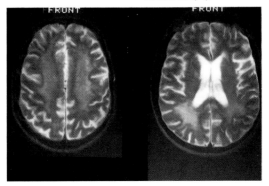

Fig. 178 AIDS-related dementia. An MRI scan showing marked cortical atrophy.

33 / Headache

Headache and facial pain may be due to serious disease, e.g. raised intracranial pressure, meningitis, giant cell arteritis (Fig. 179) and trigeminal neuralgia (Fig. 180), or to abnormalities within the eyes, ears, sinuses (Fig. 181) and teeth. Most headaches are benign and fall into one of three categories: tension, migraine and migrainous neuralgia. The most common headache is a mixture of the tension and migraine varieties.

Clinical types

Tension. Generalized headache, often starting occipitally radiating over the vertex and around the head either in a tight band or as a heavy pressure. It can be nearly continuous and present for long periods of time, often years. Blurred vision and dizziness often coexist.

Migraine. Characterized by headache attacks lasting a few hours to a day. Initial onset is usually in adolescence. There is a bilateral throbbing fronto-temporal ache associated with nausea, photophobia, phonophobia and irritability. More common in women; often there is a positive family history. In classic attacks pain tends to be one-sided and preceded by visual teichopsia/photopsia or limb tingling.

Cluster headache. Characterized by clusters of very severe pain in and around one eye and cheek. Typically attacks last 20–30 min, occur once or twice daily (often at night) over a period of weeks, and are associated with reddening/watering of the eye. More common in men; precipitated by alcohol.

Tension. Reassurance is often enough. Physical therapies such as hot and cold packs, facial vibration, physiotherapy, chiropractics, osteopathy or acupuncture are more helpful than patent analgesics.

Management

Migraine. Acute attacks should be treated with domperidone or metoclopramide and aspirin. When attacks are frequent, choose pizotifen, propranolol or amitriptyline. Imigram is effective.

Cluster headache. Treat acute attacks with ergotamine or imigram.

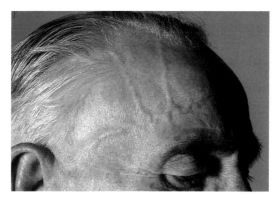

Fig. 179 Swollen, tender and non-pulsatile superficial temporal artery in giant cell arteritis.

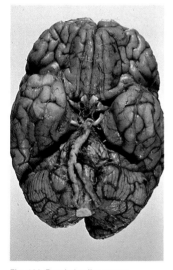

Fig. 180 Ectatic basilar artery, sometimes the cause of trigeminal neuralgia.

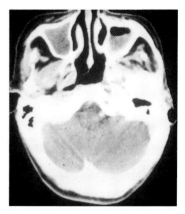

Fig. 181 CT brain scan showing bilateral antral opacification with air/fluid level on left.

Definition By dizziness, most patients mean either vertigo or a feeling of light-headedness. With vertigo, there must be a sense of motion either of self or of the environment. Once the causes of presyncope have been excluded, the complaint of light-headedness alone rarely turns up serious neurological disease.

Aetiology Vertigo, when associated with deafness, usually indicates Ménière's disease or an acoustic neuroma. Other peripheral causes of vertigo alone include acute vestibular neuronitis and benign paroxysmal positional vertigo (BPPV). Central causes of vertigo include brainstem stroke (Fig. 182), vertebrobasilar migraine, multiple sclerosis and brainstem tumours. In central cases there are usually other signs to aid localization. Very occasionally vertigo may occur as an aura in temporal lobe epilepsy (TLE).

Light-headedness (presyncope) due to postural hypotension usually occurs over some minutes and is associated with visual dimming and fading of hearing. In cardiac dysrhythmias and in carotid sinus hypersensitivity, syncope evolves much more rapidly. The most common cause of light-headedness is hyperventilation where the clue is circumoral and digital tingling.

Clinical tests To diagnose BPPV, reposition the patient from the sitting to lying position with neck extended and head turned to one side. Look for nystagmus and the reproduction of vertigo (Fig. 183). Other tests include:
- ECG (Fig. 184) and 24 h ECG monitoring
- audiometry and caloric testing
- brainstem auditory evoked potentials
- CT or MRI imaging with special emphasis on the skull base and internal auditory meati.

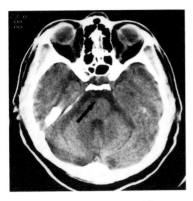

Fig. 182 CT brain scan showing right pontine infarct (arrow).

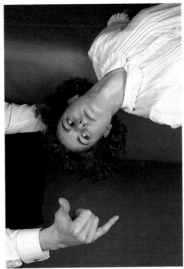

Fig. 183 Positioning of patient to look for nystagmus.

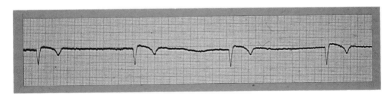

Fig. 184 Complete heart block with ventricular rate of 24 beats per min.

Disorders of stance and gait are common. They are a source of disability and of injury from accidents and falls. Gait depends on the skeleton and joints to provide stability and fulcrum, muscles to provide power and the nervous system to provide control, including sensory input, a central processing and integrating system, and an efferent system to instruct the muscles.

Aetiology

Disorders of gait may have orthopaedic, muscular, or neurological causes. Neurological causes include:
- large fibre sensory neuropathy, with loss of joint position sense
- dorsal column degeneration, e.g. vitamin B_{12} deficiency, multiple sclerosis, occult carcinoma of bronchus, hepatic disease
- tabes dorsalis
- inner ear disease, e.g. epidemic labyrinthitis (benign positional vertigo)
- brainstem disease involving vestibular nucleus and its connections
- spastic gait disorders
- cerebellar gait disorders
- frontal gait disorders
- Parkinson's disease and other extra-pyramidal gait disorders
- drug effects
- falls in the elderly; these are of multiple causation.

Clinical features

Spastic gait disorder (Fig. 185) is characterized by a narrow-based, short-stepped, lurching gait, with poor elevation of toe and forefoot, so that the toes seem to catch on the ground. The patient is relatively well balanced, and may be able to hobble into a short-stepped run. ➡

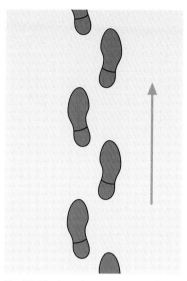

Fig. 185 The foot placement pattern of spastic gait disorder. Note the narrow base and the short steps.

Cerebellar gait disorder causes a wide-based gait of irregular cadence with a tendency to fall, especially when turning. There is a wandering quality to the progression in any direction caused by the irregularity in length, direction and rhythm of the steps. The gait of acute alcohol intoxication is a well-known example (Fig. 186).

Parkinsonian gait disorder (Fig. 187) has an accelerating quality, with small steps, a rigidity of posture in a flexed stance, and an inability to change rhythm or frequency of the gait pattern.

Frontal gait disorder is associated with a 'magnetic' attraction of the feet to the ground, short, rapid, shuffling steps and freezing in mid-task. There is often marked disequilibrium.

Myopathic gait disorder shows bilateral hip weakness with Trendelenberg floppiness of hip posture, and an exaggerated lumbar lordosis.

Peripheral neuropathy causes a high steppage gait because there is distal weakness causing foot drop.

Tabes dorsalis and other sensory disorders cause a stamping high steppage gait, caused by the requirement to increase sensory input by striking the feet hard on the ground.

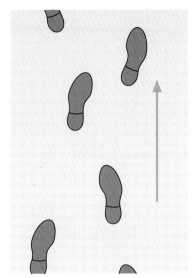

Fig. 186 The foot placement pattern of cerebellar. The foot placement pattern is wide-based and irregular, resembling the pattern of cerebellar disease. In sensory neuropathy the disorder is markedly worsened by eye closure, which removes visual cues upon which the patient is reliant.

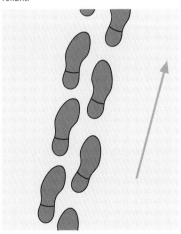

Fig. 187 The foot placement pattern of Parkinson's disease. Note the short overlapping gait cadence.

Index